ECONOMIC ISSUES, PROBLEMS AND PERSPECTIVES

ECONOMIC CONDITIONS IMPACT ON PARTICIPATION IN NUTRITION ASSISTANCE PROGRAMS

ECONOMIC ISSUES, PROBLEMS AND PERSPECTIVES

Additional books in this series can be found on Nova's website under the Series tab.

Additional E-books in this series can be found on Nova's website under the E-book tab.

NUTRITION AND DIET RESEARCH PROGRESS

Additional books in this series can be found on Nova's website under the Series tab.

Additional E-books in this series can be found on Nova's website under the E-book tab.

ECONOMIC ISSUES, PROBLEMS AND PERSPECTIVES

ECONOMIC CONDITIONS IMPACT ON PARTICIPATION IN NUTRITION ASSISTANCE PROGRAMS

OSCAR GUTIERREZ
EDITOR

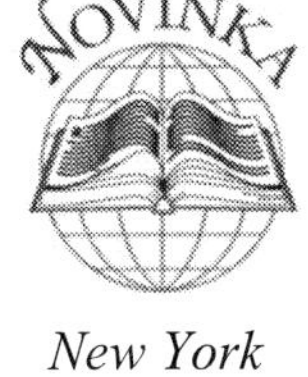

New York

For permission to use material from this book please contact us:
Telephone 631-231-7269; Fax 631-231-8175
Web Site: http://www.novapublishers.com

Additional color graphics may be available in the e-book version of this book.

Library of Congress Cataloging-in-Publication Data

ISBN: 978-1-62417-520-6

Published by Nova Science Publishers, Inc. † New York

CONTENTS

PREFACE

The U.S. Department of Agriculture (USDA) administers 15 domestic nutrition assistance programs. The five largest programs are: the Supplemental Nutrition Assistance Program (SNAP, formerly the Food Stamp Program), Special Supplemental Nutrition Program for Women, Infants, and Children (WIC), National School Lunch Program (NSLP), School Breakfast Program (SBP), and Child and Adult Care Food Program (CACFP). Although SNAP's reputation as one of the Nation's primary counter-cyclical assistance program, expanding during economic downturns and contracting during periods of economic growth, is well established, there has been little analysis of the effect of the economy on other programs. This book examines the relationship between U.S. economic conditions and participation in the U.S. Department of Agriculture's nutrition assistance programs and how changes in program policy may have influenced this relationship.

Chapter 1 - This study, based on 1976-2010 data, examines the relationship between U.S. economic conditions and participation in the U.S. Department of Agriculture's five largest nutrition assistance programs. It also describes how changes in program policy and other factors may have influenced this relationship. The five programs are: Supplemental Nutrition Assistance Program (SNAP, formerly the Food Stamp Program), Special Supplemental Nutrition Program for Women, Infants, and Children (WIC), National School Lunch Program (NSLP), School Breakfast Program (SBP), and Child and Adult Care Food Program (CACFP). Although SNAP's reputation as one of the Nation's primary counter- cyclical assistance programs—expanding during economic downturns and contracting during periods of economic growth—is well established, there has been little analysis of the effect of the economy on the other programs. The results of this study strongly suggest that, to varying degrees, economic conditions influence participation in all the major nutrition assistance programs, not just in SNAP.

Chapter 2 - Over the years, Congress has authorized and the federal government has administered programs to provide food to the hungry and to other vulnerable populations in this country. This report offers a brief overview of hunger and food insecurity along with the related network of programs. The report is structured around three main tables that contain information about each program, including its authorizing language, administering agency, eligibility, services provided, participation data, and funding information. In between the tables, contextual information about this policy area and program administration is provided that may assist Congress in tracking developments in domestic food assistance. This report provides a bird's-eye view of domestic food assistance and can be used both to learn about the details of individual programs as well as compare and contrast features across programs.

This report includes overview information for the U.S. Department of Agriculture's Food and Nutrition Service (USDA-FNS) Programs as well as nutrition programs administered by the U.S. Department of Health and Human Services' Administration on Aging (HHS-AOA). USDA-FNS programs include nutrition programs authorized in the 2008 farm bill (the Food, Conservation, and Energy Act of 2008; P.L. 110-246). Programs included in the farm bill are the Supplemental Nutrition Assistance Program (SNAP), Emergency Food Assistance Program (TEFAP), Commodity Supplemental Food Program (CSFP), Fresh Fruit and Vegetable Program, and the Senior Farmers' Market Nutrition Program. USDA-FNS also administers programs not contained in the farm bill: the Special Supplemental Nutrition Program for Women, Infants, and Children (WIC) and Child Nutrition programs (School Breakfast Program, National School Lunch Program (NSLP), Summer Food Service Program (SFSP), Special Milk Program, and Child and Adult Care Food Program (CACFP)). HHS-AOA programs are the nutrition programs contained in the Older Americans Act (OAA)—Congregate Nutrition Program; Home Delivered Nutrition Program; Grants to Native Americans: Supportive and Nutrition Services; and the Nutrition Service Incentive Program (NSIP).

In: Economic Conditions ...
Editor: Oscar Gutierrez

ISBN: 978-1-62417-520-6

Chapter 1

HOW ECONOMIC CONDITIONS AFFECT PARTICIPATION IN USDA NUTRITION ASSISTANCE PROGRAMS*

Kenneth Hanson and Victor Oliveira

ABSTRACT

This study, based on 1976-2010 data, examines the relationship between U.S. economic conditions and participation in the U.S. Department of Agriculture's five largest nutrition assistance programs. It also describes how changes in program policy and other factors may have influenced this relationship. The five programs are: Supplemental Nutrition Assistance Program (SNAP, formerly the Food Stamp Program), Special Supplemental Nutrition Program for Women, Infants, and Children (WIC), National School Lunch Program (NSLP), School Breakfast Program (SBP), and Child and Adult Care Food Program (CACFP). Although SNAP's reputation as one of the Nation's primary counter- cyclical assistance programs—expanding during economic downturns and contracting during periods of economic growth—is well established, there has been little analysis of the effect of the economy on the other programs. The results of this study strongly suggest that, to varying degrees, economic conditions influence participation in all the major nutrition assistance programs, not just in SNAP.

* This is an edited, reformatted and augmented version of a United States Department of Agriculture publication, dated September 2012.

Keywords: Nutrition assistance programs, business cycle, caseloads, participation, unemployment rate, Supplemental Nutrition Assistance Program (SNAP), Special Supplemental Nutrition Program for Women, Infants, and Children (WIC), National School Lunch Program (NSLP), School Breakfast Program (SBP), and Child and Adult Care Food Program (CACFP)

SUMMARY

What Is the Issue?

The U.S. Department of Agriculture (USDA) administers 15 domestic nutrition assistance programs. The five largest programs—Supplemental Nutrition Assistance Program (SNAP, formerly the Food Stamp Program), Special Supplemental Nutrition Program for Women, Infants, and Children (WIC), National School Lunch Program (NSLP), School Breakfast Program (SBP), and Child and Adult Care Food Program (CACFP)—accounted for 96 percent of USDA's expenditures for nutrition assistance in fiscal 2010. These programs form a nutritional safety net for millions of children and low- income adults, a role that is especially important when the economy falters and many Americans lose jobs and income.

SNAP's reputation as one of the Nation's primary countercyclical assistance programs—expanding during economic downturns and contracting during periods of economic growth—is well established. However, there has been little analysis of the effect of the economy on the other programs. This is the first study to investigate the relationship between economic conditions and participation at the national level across USDA's five largest nutrition assistance programs. The report also provides a detailed description of how changes in program policies and other factors such as demographics affected participation, augmenting or offsetting business cycle effects.

What Did the Study Find?

The results of this study suggest that, to varying degrees, economic conditions, as measured by the unemployment rate, influence participation in all the major nutrition assistance programs, not just in SNAP.

Key findings include the following:

- The increase in SNAP participation during the 2008-10 period of economic decline (which included the recent recession) was consistent with the increase during previous periods of economic decline, at 2 to 3 million participants per 1-percentage-point increase in the unemployment rate.
- Policy changes pertaining to eligibility rules, benefit levels, outreach, and the application-certification process tended to augment the increase in SNAP participation due to economic conditions in each period of economic decline.
- Before being fully funded in the late 1990s, WIC participation was rationed by the program's budgetary limits and expanded as the budget grew. The introduction of infant formula rebates in the late 1980s lowered the cost of the WIC food package, enabling more people to participate within the program's budget and fueling an increase in the annual average growth in participation.
- After reaching full funding in the late 1990s, WIC caseloads became more sensitive to economic conditions, increasing (decreasing) by nearly 2.5 percent (200,000 participants) per 1-percentage-point increase (decrease) in the unemployment rate. The number of births also had a strong influence on the number of participants; for instance, during the recession of 2008-09, the low number of births tended to counter the growth in participation prompted by economic conditions.
- The percentage of participants receiving free and reduced-price meals in the child nutrition programs (NSLP, SBP, and CACFP) appears related to economic conditions, rising with the unemployment rate during periods of economic decline.
- Total participation in the child nutrition programs has steadily increased during periods of both economic growth and decline. These programs serve both low- and high-income children.
- NSLP participation appears to be linked to school enrollment, while availability of the program in schools has been a key to the growth of SBP participation.

How Was the Study Conducted?

The study used national-level administrative data on program participation collected by USDA's Food and Nutrition Service (FNS) and data on unemployment rates published by the Bureau of Labor Statistics. The study period—fiscal year 1976 to fiscal year 2010—encompassed four complete business cycles, each consisting of a period of economic growth characterized by a falling unemployment rate and a period of economic decline characterized by a rising unemployment rate. For each period of growth and decline, the authors examined the relationship between the fluctuation in program participation and the unemployment rate. They also examined various publications and regulations to determine how program policy and other factors (such as demographics) may have influenced the relationship between program participation and the unemployment rate.

INTRODUCTION

The U.S. Department of Agriculture (USDA) administers 15 domestic nutri- tion assistance programs that form a nutrition safety net for millions of children and low-income adults, a role that is especially important when the economy falters and many Americans lose jobs and income. As means- tested programs, the size of the eligible population is intrinsically linked to the economy.

That is, the number of those who are eligible rises during recessionary periods when the number of unemployed and poor people increases and falls during periods of economic growth as conditions improve. The extent to which participation in these programs responds to changing economic conditions affects not only the lives of millions of Americans, but has Federal budgetary implications as well.

This is the first study to investigate the relationship between economic condi- tions and participation at the national level across USDA's five largest nutri- tion assistance programs.

The report also provides a detailed description of how changes in program policy and other factors—e.g., demographics—may have affected participation and thus influenced the relationship between program participation and economic conditions. The study period, from fiscal year (FY) 1976 to FY 2010, covers much of each program's history, while encompassing the growth and decline phases of four business cycles.[1] By including the recession of 2008-09 (often called the Great Recession), we are able to compare how the change in participation relative to the change in economic conditions during that period compares with participation changes during previous economic downturns.

The five programs examined in this report—Supplemental Nutrition Assistance Program (SNAP, formerly the Food Stamp Program); Special Supplemental Nutrition Program for Women, Infants, and Children (WIC); National School Lunch Program (NSLP); School Breakfast Program (SBP); and Child and Adult Care Food Program (CACFP)—accounted for 96 percent of USDA's expenditures for nutrition assistance in fiscal 2010 (Oliveira, 2011). The programs vary by target population, eligibility require- ments, form of benefit provided, funding mechanism, age of recipients, and size (i.e., in terms of both number of participants and expenditures) (table 1).

As illustrated in figure 1, the relationship between program caseloads and changing economic conditions—as measured by the unemployment rate—varies across the programs. SNAP caseloads clearly follow the unemploy- ment rate, supporting SNAP's reputation as one of the Nation's primary countercyclical assistance programs, expanding during economic downturns and contracting during periods of economic growth. At first glance, there is no apparent relationship between program caseloads and economic condi- tions for the other programs. For example, SNAP is the only program whose participation appears to spike during the recent economic downturn after 2008. The seeming nonresponse of these other programs raised the primary question motivating this study: Do changes in economic conditions affect only participation in SNAP or also participation in the other major nutrition assistance programs?

A number of studies have documented the relationship between economic conditions and participation in SNAP (e.g., Klerman and Danielson, 2011). These studies found a positive effect of the unemployment rate on SNAP case-loads, while also taking into account the impact of policies and other factors that were in effect during the study periods (appendix A provides a brief review of these studies). Each study focused on specific policies that covered relatively short periods, while this report compares the relationship of SNAP participa-tion with the unemployment rate over four business cycles (eight periods of economic growth and decline) that occurred during 1976 to 2010.

There has been little to no analysis of the relationship between participation and the economy for the other nutrition assistance programs. The few studies that have analyzed the effect of the economy on WIC reached contradictory conclusions. Bitler et al. (2003), using data from 1992 to 2000, found that WIC participation was not strongly correlated with unemployment, while Swann (2010) found a positive correlation between unemployment and WIC participation for 1983 to 2006. No recent studies have examined the econo- my's impact on the child nutrition programs.

Table 1. Selected characteristics of the major USDA nutrition assistance programs

Program	Year permanently authorized	Target popula-tion	Income eligibility limit	Form of benefit provided	Funding mechanism	Average participation in FY 2010	Total USDA expenditures in FY 2010
SNAP	1964	Households	130 percent of poverty	Electronic benefits to purchase food	Entitlement program	40.3 million participants per month	$68.3 billion
WIC	1974	Women, infants, and children	185 percent of poverty	Supplemental foods	Discretionary program	9.2 million participants per month	$6.7 billion
NSLP	1946	Primary and secondary students	130 percent of poverty for free meals and 185 percent of poverty for reduced-price meals[1]	Lunch	Entitlement program	31.7 million children per day	$10.9 billion
SBP	1975	Primary and secondary students	130 percent of poverty for free meals and 185 percent of poverty for reduced-price meals[1]	Breakfast	Entitlement program	11.7 million children per day	$2.9 billion
CACFP	1978	Children and adults in day care	No limit	Breakfast, lunch, dinner, and snacks	Entitlement program	3.4 million persons per day	$2.6 billion

Source: USDA Economic Research Service calculations based on USDA Food and Nutrition Service data. Participation and expenditure data are from the USDA Food and Nutrition Service program data Webpage as of April 30, 2012.

Note: SNAP= Supplemental Nutrition Assistance Program; WIC = Special Supplemental Nutrition Program for Women, Infants, and Children; NSLP= National School Lunch Program; SBP= School Breakfast Program; CACFP= Child and Adult Care Food Program.

[1] However, all children attending schools that offer NSLP or SBP may participate in these programs. If the household's income exceeds the maximum limit for free and reduced-price meals, the student can purchase a "full price" meal (i.e., a paid-for meal).

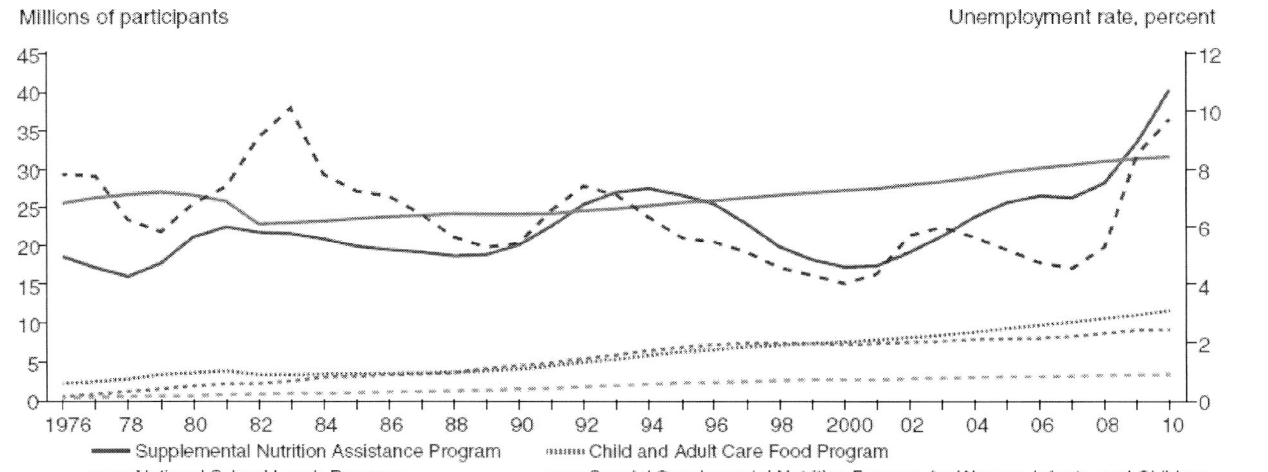

Source: USDA Food and Nutrition Service data and U.S. Department of Labor, Bureau of Labor Statistics data.

Figure 1. Nutrition assistance program participation and unemployment rate, fiscal years 1976-2010.

As a descriptive study, this analysis does not quantify the relative effects of the economy, program policies, and other factors on program participation. Rather, it is an exploratory examination of whether participation in all of the major nutrition assistance programs, and not just SNAP, are related to economic conditions.

The study's major contribution is that it suggests that economic conditions, to varying degrees, influence program participation in all the major nutri-tion assistance programs, not just SNAP. For example, WIC caseloads appear to have become more responsive to economic conditions after the program became fully funded in the late 1990s. While economic conditions do not affect total participation in the child nutrition programs (NSLP, SBP, and CACFP), they do appear to affect the proportion of participants receiving free or reduced-price meals. Thus, these other programs, like SNAP, are countercyclical, with their use by needy families increasing during economic downturns. These findings lay the groundwork for future statistical analyses of the relationship between program participation and economic conditions for the non-SNAP programs.

The next chapter describes the data and methodology underlying this study. This is followed by the descriptive analysis of the relationship between program participation and economic conditions and the influence that changes in program policy and other factors have had on this relationship.

Each program is discussed in a separate chapter, allowing readers to focus on those programs of interest to them. Although the relationship between SNAP participation and economic conditions is well established, it is included as a separate chapter for comparison with the other programs.

Data and Methodology

To examine the relationship between economic conditions and participation in the various programs, this report uses national-level administrative data on program participation from FY 1976 to FY 2010 from USDA's Food and Nutrition Service (USDA-FNS), the agency responsible for managing the programs.[2] Program participation for SNAP and WIC refers to the annual average number of monthly participants, that is, monthly participation aver- aged over the 12 months of a fiscal year (October to September).[3] Program participation for NSLP and SBP refers to average daily participation averaged over 9 months of a school year (September through May). For CACFP, the annual average participation data represent average daily attendance over the fiscal year. The fiscal year and school year notations in this report are omitted and referred to as annual data.

The study period from 1976 to 2010 includes four complete business cycles, each consisting of a period of economic growth and a period of economic decline (fig. 2). For this report, the economic periods were determined by one of the Nation's primary economic indicators, the official unemploy- ment rate published by the U.S. Department of Labor's Bureau of Labor Statistics. Fiscal year annual unemployment rates were calculated as an annual average of seasonally adjusted monthly unemployment rates. Periods of economic growth were characterized by a falling unemployment rate and periods of economic decline by a rising unemployment rate. Holding other factors constant, program participation is expected to increase during periods of economic decline—reflecting increased need and eligibility for nutri-tion assistance—and decrease during periods of economic growth (see box, "Unemployment Rate and Poverty Rate Over the Business Cycle," p. 5).

The years in which each period of economic growth and decline started and ended were specified by whether the year-to-year change in the unemploy-ment rate was negative or positive. The dates for the periods of economic growth and decline are listed in table 2, along with the annual average percentage-point change in the unemployment rate. The periods of economic decline capture each of the recessions that occurred over the years of the analysis (fig. 2).[4]

However, the starting and ending dates for the periods of economic decline often extend beyond the official dates of the recession. That is, the unemployment rate often started to rise before the recession's starting date and continued to rise—for a year or more—after the recession's ending date. Unemployment rates often do not decline until after a recession has offi- cially ended, in part because businesses do not begin to hire until there is a clear indication that the economy is improving. Businesses in some industries are able to increase production without hiring more workers during the initial phase of recovery by increasing production per unit of labor when capacity utilization is low (Schreft et al., 2005).

To examine the relationship between program participation and economic conditions across the various periods of economic growth and decline (busi-ness cycles), the annual average change in participation—expressed both as number of participants and as percentage of participants—was calculated for each period.

The annual average change was calculated for each period by first calculating the year-to-year difference (and percentage change) in the annual average number of participants, and then taking the average of these year-to-year differences (and percentage changes) over the years in each of the periods. Since the number of years in each period is unequal, the change in participation and the unemployment rate during each period are calculated as annual average changes over the period, which makes for better comparability across periods. For the child nutrition programs (NSLP, SBP, and CACFP), the annual average percentage change in the percentage of participants receiving free and reduced-price meals was also calculated. Because the *number* of participants receiving free and reduced-price meals increased each year with the growth in school enrollment, the *percentage* of participants receiving free and reduced-price meals is a better indicator for measuring the influence of economic conditions. To keep the analysis as straightforward as possible, participation figures cited in this report have not been normalized by population and reflect the actual number of participants. Population growth was generally steady over the study period, averaging 1 percent per year while ranging from 0.7 percent to 1.3 percent (U.S. Bureau of Census, annual population data). The impact of population growth on participation (including related issues such as trends in births and school enrollment) varied across programs and is discussed, when relevant, in the appropriate chapters.

Unemployment Rate and Poverty Rate Over the Business Cycle

A number of indicators provide information about the overall state of the economy, such as Gross Domestic Product (GDP), real income, wholesale-retail sales, industrial production, employment, and the unemployment rate. Unlike many of these measures, the unemployment rate has a more direct relationship with the poverty rate, which is a measure of household hardship and economic well-being and underlies the need for nutrition assistance. Figure 2 shows the relationship between the unemployment rate and poverty rate over the periods of economic growth and decline between 1976 and 2010. The year-to-year change in the poverty rate and unemployment rate has a correlation coefficient of 0.76 over these years, suggesting that a change in the unemployment rate is a good proxy for a change in the poverty rate. This study used the unemployment rate to represent economic conditions. Unemployment is a well-recognized indicator of the state of the economy, published monthly with only a 1-month lag and used by the Federal Government as a forecast variable in budgetary projections of nutrition assistance program caseloads.

While the Bureau of Labor Statistics publishes five alternative unemployment rates in addition to the "official" one, for national annual data the various measures of unemployment are highly correlated, and so the official unemployment rate is used in our analysis. We use the unemployment rate rather than the number of unemployed because of greater public familiarity with the rate. An exception to the high correlation between the unemployment rate and the poverty rate occurred during the 2004-07 period of economic growth. While the unemployment rate fell throughout this period, the poverty rate rose in 2004, fell slightly during the next 2 years, and then rose again in 2007 for a net change of zero over the period. The deviation in the trend between unemployment and poverty rates during this period suggests that while the economy was growing and the unemployment rate was falling, the economic well-being of many households did not improve. Previous research has suggested that labor market conditions for less skilled workers, such as real wages and job opportunities, did not improve as much or as quickly as they had during past economic recoveries and poverty rates remained close to those of the previous period of economic decline (Bivens and Irons, 2008; Blank, 2009; Greenstone and Looney, 2011).

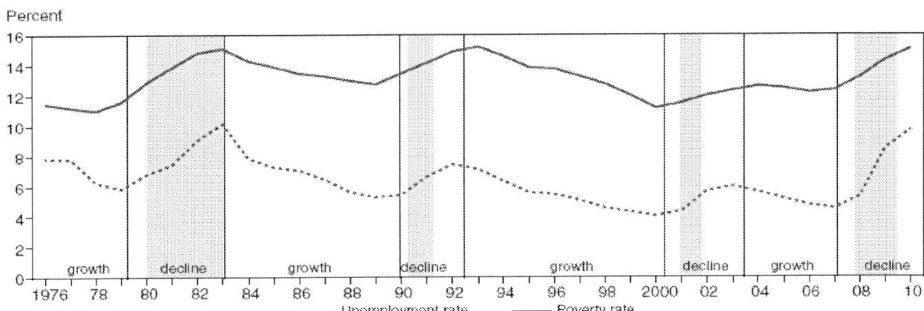

Source: USDA Food and Nutrition Service data, U.S. Department of Labor, Bureau of Labor Statistics data, and U.S. Census Bureau data.

Note: The bars distinguish periods of growth and decline as defined by fiscal year annual unemployment rates (calculated as an annual average of the official monthly unemployment rates published by the U.S. Department of Labor's Bureau of Labor Statistics). Periods of economic growth were characterized by a falling unemployment rate and periods of economic decline by a rising unemployment rate. Shaded areas represent National Bureau of Economic Research periods of recession.

Figure 2. Unemployment rate and poverty rate in periods of economic growth and decline, fiscal years 1976-2010.

Table 2. Periods of economic growth and decline and change in unemployment rate

Fiscal years	Economic period	Annual average percentage-point change in unemployment rate	Duration of period in fiscal years
1976-1979	growth	-0.55	4
1980-1983	decline	1.07	4
1984-1989	growth	-0.81	6
1990-1992	decline	0.72	3
1993-2000	growth	-0.43	8
2001-2003	decline	0.66	3
2004-2007	growth	-0.37	4
2008-2010	decline	1.74	3

The size of change in the unemployment rate varied across the different periods of growth and decline (table 2). For example, the largest annual average percentage-point change in the unemployment rate occurred during the 2008-10 period of economic decline, which included the Great Recession, at an annual average of 1.74 percentage points per year. Thus, changes in program participation are not expected to be equal across the various periods. To better compare the relationship between program participation and the unemployment rate during the 2008-10 period with that of other economic periods, the annual average change in program participation during each period of growth and decline was divided by the annual average percentage point change in the unemployment rate that occurred during the period. This normalized the change in participation to a 1-percentage-point change in the unemployment rate, improving the comparability of the participation/unemployment relationship across periods. For all the programs, changes in program policy and other factors have affected participation and thus influenced the relationship between program participation and the unemployment rate. In general, the direction of the effect on participation from these changes is evident, but not the magnitude of the effect. In some cases, changes in program policy and other factors augment the response of program participation to economic conditions; in other cases, they dampen or even negate the effect of changing economic conditions. Changes in program policy can occur through legislative changes and changes in administrative practices pertaining to such factors as eligi- bility rules, benefit levels, application-certification process (i.e., accessi- bility), and outreach. Other factors, such as funding levels (WIC), program availability (child nutrition programs), demographics (WIC), and economic factors other than the unemployment rate (such as wages for low-skilled workers) may also affect program participation. This report describes key changes in program policy and other factors and notes whether they would have augmented or dampened the effect of changes to the unemployment rate on participation.

SUPPLEMENTAL NUTRITION ASSISTANCE PROGRAM (SNAP)

SNAP—formerly the Food Stamp Program—is the cornerstone of USDA's nutrition assistance programs, accounting for 72 percent of all Federal nutrition assistance spending in fiscal 2010 (Oliveira, 2011). By providing electronic benefits that can be used like cash for food purchases at most grocery stores, SNAP enables participants—half of whom are children—to improve their diets by increasing their food-purchasing power. Benefit levels depend on household income and size. As a household's income increases, SNAP benefits decrease. Unlike other nutrition assistance programs that are targeted toward special population groups, SNAP is available to most needy households, subject to certain work and immigration-status require- ments. To be eligible for SNAP, the gross monthly income of households must be 130 percent or less of the Federal poverty guidelines (households with an elderly or disabled member are excluded from the gross income test). Net monthly income must be 100 percent or less of Federal poverty guidelines, where net income equals gross income minus a standard deduc- tion, a housing expense deduction, earned income deduction, child care deduction, and several other smaller deductions.

As illustrated in figure 3, SNAP caseloads and the unemployment rate gener- ally trend together, with participation increasing during economic downturns and decreasing during periods of economic growth. Over the full 1976-2010 period, the correlation coefficient between year-to-year change in the unem- ployment rate and year-to-year change in SNAP participation was 0.60; after omitting the earlier years from 1976-83 when policy changes had an espe- cially large impact on participation, the correlation coefficient rises to 0.70.[5] The relationship between SNAP participation and the unemployment rate has been well established in a number of empirical studies (see appendix A for a review of this literature). An advantage of these studies is that they estimate the impact of economic conditions on program participation while simultaneously estimating the impact of program policy. However, most of the studies omitted national policies and relied on variation in State economic conditions and implementation of program policy to estimate their models and were only able to explain about 50 percent of the change in participation (Klerman and Danielson, 2011; Mabli et al., 2009).This chapter provides a broad, historical context for assessing how economic conditions and program policy have influenced SNAP participation over a long period. Specifically, it describes and compares the relationship of SNAP participation with the unemployment rate over four business cycles (eight periods of economic growth and decline) that occurred during the study period of 1976 to 2010 and describes how numerous changes in program policy influenced this relationship (fig. 4). Sometimes the change in policy augmented the influence of the unemployment rate on participation, while at other times the change in policy dampened the influence of the unemploy- ment rate on participation. During the first period of analysis in this report, the 1976-79 period of economic growth, there was a slight annual average increase in SNAP participation, a result contrary to expectations (fig. 5 and appendix B, table 1). SNAP participation increased in 1976, a continuation of the increase during the economic decline of 1974-75 (prior to the period of analysis in this study). This could have resulted from a continued nationwide expansion of program participation once all State and localities started making SNAP available in 1974 and from a possible lag in the economic gains to low-income households during the initial period of an economic recovery (see box, “Asymmetrical Lags in SNAP Participation,” p. 11). SNAP participation finally decreased in 1977 and 1978 along with the unemployment rate, as would be expected. However, SNAP participation increased once again in 1979 as a result of the Food Stamp Act of 1977 (P.L. 95-113) that made major changes to the program (Wertheimer and Fletcher, 1985; Dynaski et al., 1991). A key change was elimination of the purchase requirement (U.S. Department of Agriculture, 2011a). Prior to the Act, program participants were required to purchase food stamps at a discounted price that depended on household income.[6] The purchase requirement limited participation among the very poor because people with little available cash found it difficult to purchase the food stamps (Ohls and Beebout, 1993). The Act was enacted near the end of 1977, and States were given a year to implement the revisions, so the impact of the 1977 legislation on program participation would not have been felt until 1979. An increase in the poverty rate from 1978 to 1979, reflecting increased economic need, would also have been associated with an increase in partici- pation (Wertheimer and Fletcher, 1985).

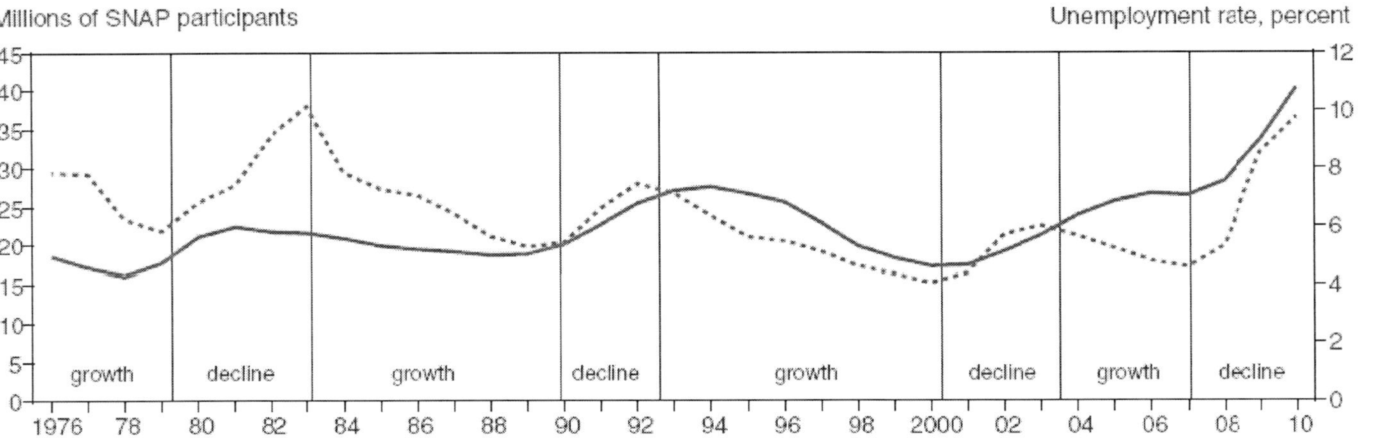

Source: USDA Food and Nutrition Service data and U.S. Department of Labor, Bureau of Labor Statistics data.

Figure 3. Supplemental Nutrition Assistance Program (SNAP) participation and unemployment rate, fiscal years 1976-2010.

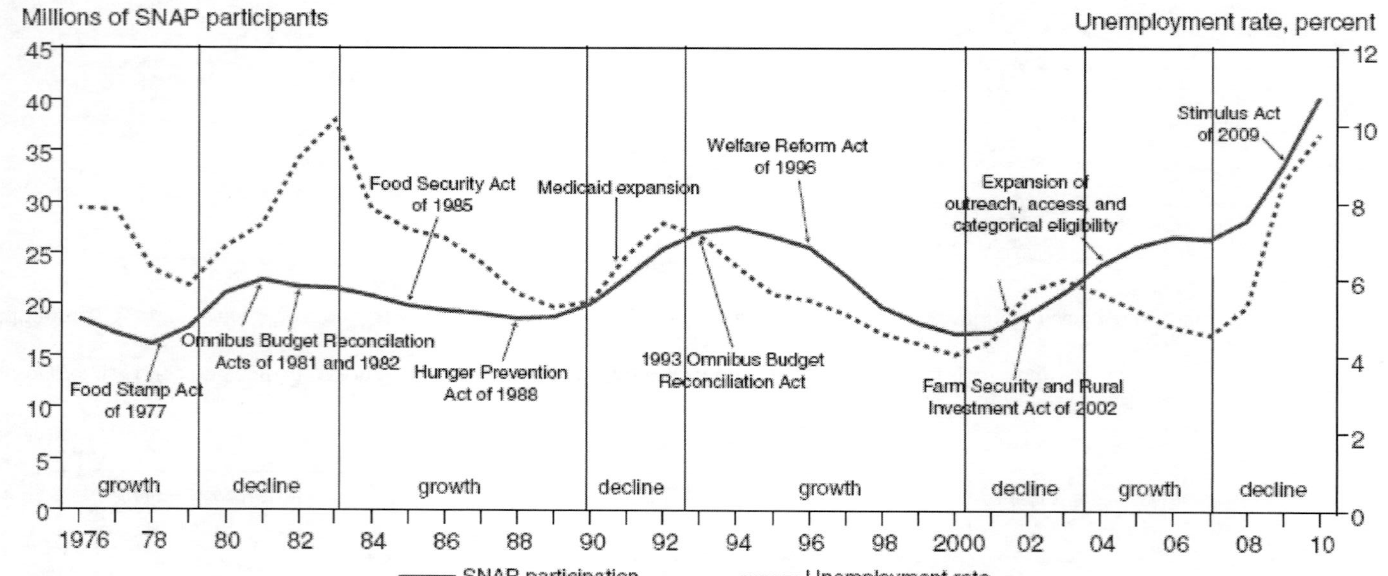

Source: Based on USDA Food and Nutrition Service information.

Figure 4. Policies and legislative acts impacting Supplemental Nutrition Assistance Program (SNAP) participation, fiscal years 1976-2010.

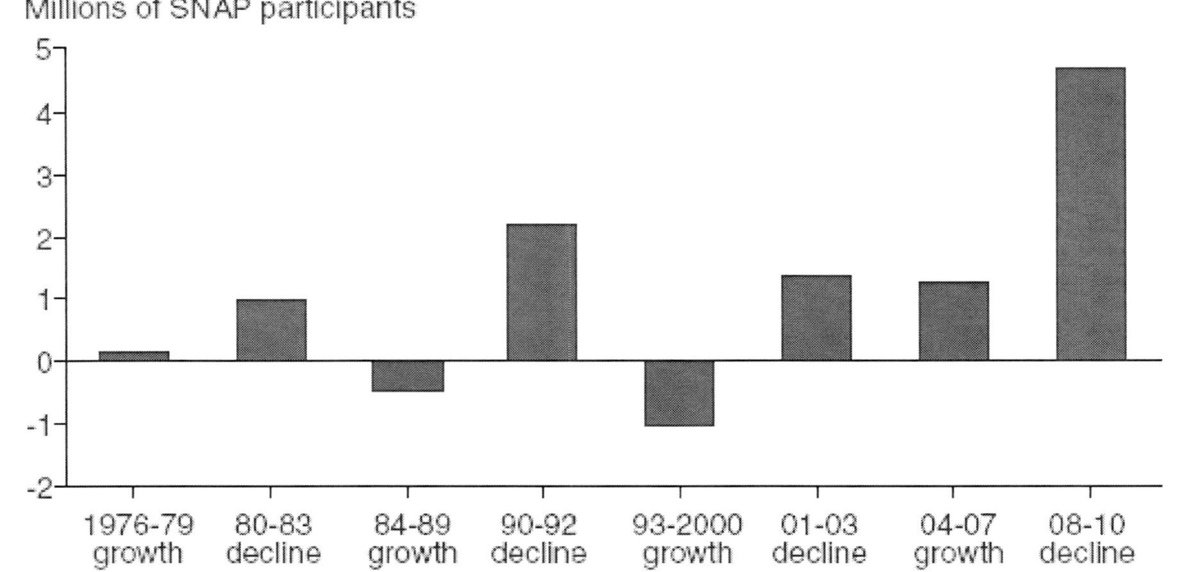

Source: USDA Economic Research Service, based on USDA Food and Nutrition Service data.

Figure 5. Supplemental Nutrition Assistance Program (SNAP) participation, annual average change during periods of economic growth (blue) and decline (red).

Over the 1980-83 period of economic decline, SNAP participation increased by an average 5.6 percent (1.0 million participants) per year (fig. 5), but the direction of change varied during the period. SNAP participation increased by an average 12.9 percent (2.4 million participants) per year during the first 2 years of this period (appendix B, table 1), a likely result of the economic decline and a continued response to the 1977 legislation.

During the last 2 years of the period, however, SNAP participation fell by an average 1.8 percent (402,000 participants) per year, even as the unemployment rate continued to rise.

The Omnibus Budget Reconciliation Acts of 1981 and 1982 (P.L. 97-35 and 97-253) contributed to this contrary result (Wertheimer and Fletcher, 1985; Dynaski et al., 1991).

The Acts tightened eligibility rules, thereby reducing the number of persons eligible to participate, and reduced benefits, lowering the incentive to participate among the eligible population (see box, "SNAP Take-Up Rates," p. 12).[7]

As expected, participation fell during the 1984-89 period of economic growth. However the reduction was relatively small: an average 2.3 percent (470,000 participants) per year (fig. 5).

The Food Security Act of 1985 (P.L. 99-198) and the Hunger Prevention Act of 1988 (P.L 100-435) eased eligibility rules, made several changes to administrative rules that opened up program access, and provided greater incentives to participate by increasing the benefit amount to most recipients. These policy changes diminished the effect that the improved economic conditions would normally have had on program participation (Dynaski et al., 1991).[8]

The 1990-92 period of economic decline saw an average increase of 10.6 percent (2.2 million participants) per year in participation (fig. 5). This large increase was due to the economic decline as well as to changes in program policy that increased the take-up rate.

For instance, expansion in the Medicaid program increased the SNAP take-up rate because there was a greater effort to inform Medicaid applicants about SNAP and to encourage them to apply for benefits (McConnell, 1991).

In addition, the Hunger Prevention Act of 1988 would have continued to have an effect on program participation during this period (Dynaski et al., 1991).

Asymmetrical Lags in SNAP Participation

SNAP caseloads over the business cycles appear to exhibit asymmetrical lags in response to a change in the unemployment rate. During each of the four economic declines that occurred during the 1976-2010 study period, SNAP participation rose quickly and in step with the unemployment rate. Essentially there was no lag in the participation response to the rising unemployment rate, and in each period the rates of increase were about the same. During three of the four periods of economic growth, however, reductions in SNAP participation lagged behind decreases in the unemployment rate. That is, as the unemployment rate started to fall during the early phase of the 1976-79, 1993-2000, and 2004-07 periods of economic growth, SNAP participation continued to increase for 1 or more years. The one exception occurred during the 1984-89 period of economic growth and was likely due to the Omnibus Budget Reconciliation Acts of 1981 and 1982, which had already started a reduction in participation prior to the growth period.

One explanation for a lagged response of SNAP participation to a reduction in the unemployment rate during the early stage of an economic recovery is that labor market outcomes (such as unemployment) for less skilled workers vary more over the business cycle than do those of more skilled workers (Hoynes, 2000; Blank, 2009). The improvement of economic conditions during the early stage of recovery, when the unemployment rate finally starts to fall, takes longer to be felt by low-income workers in low-skilled jobs who are more likely to participate in SNAP. The phenomena of jobless recoveries could also contribute to asymmetry in the business cycle (Schreft et al., 2005), particularly if the low-skilled jobs are slower to recover than high-skilled jobs.

The empirical studies of SNAP participation (see appendix A) account for a lagged response in participation to a change in the unemployment rate by lagging the unemployment rate for 1 or more years in the estimated model, along with the current unemployment rate (e.g., Klerman and Danielson, 2011). However, this treatment of the lagged response is symmetrical over the business cycle and does not focus on the slow reduction in participation during the early stage of an economic recovery. There is some literature that addresses the issue of asymmetry of the unemployment rate over the business cycle that could be used to assess asymmetry of SNAP participation over the cycle (e.g., Neftci, 1984; Sichel, 1993).

SNAP Take-Up Rates

The number of participants in SNAP is affected by changes in the number of persons who are eligible to participate as well as the percentage of eligible persons who choose to participate, that is, the take-up rate (also known as the participation rate). Changes in program policy may affect the take-up rate. For example, expanded outreach and simplification of the application process pull more eligible people into SNAP, while legislation that increases (decreases) benefit levels may provide an incentive for more (or disincentive for fewer) eligible people to apply to the program. Economic conditions may also affect take-up rates by influencing eligible persons' decisions on whether to participate in the program. The figure illustrates the relationship between SNAP caseloads and two types of take-up rates over the business cycle.[1] The take-up rate for persons is the ratio of participants to eligible persons. The take-up rate for benefits compares (as a percent) the actual benefits received by participants with the benefits that would be issued if all eligible persons participated. In general, both measures of take-up rates (persons and benefits) follow the trend in total participation (i.e., caseloads). This suggests that changes in caseloads during periods of economic decline and growth are not solely due to changes in the number of eligible persons, but are also driven by a change in the take-up rate.

Trends in Supplemental Nutrition Assistance Program (SNAP). take-up rates and participation

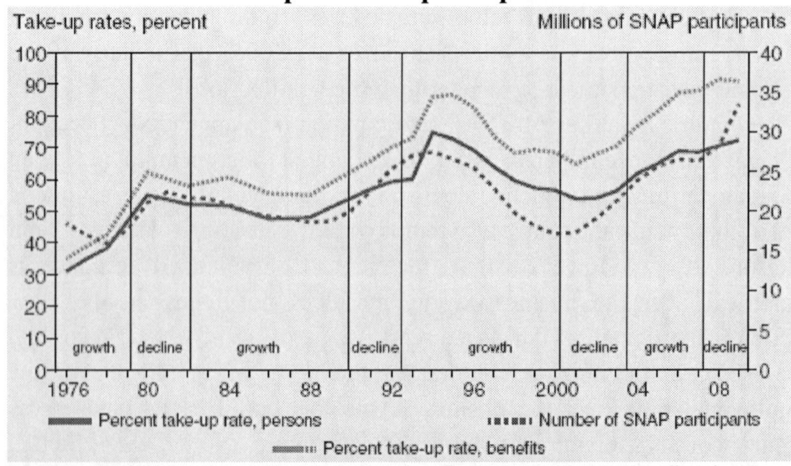

Source: USDA Food and Nutrition Service data. Years shown are fiscal years.

[1]The take-up rates were estimated using household survey data and program data on participation. There are breaks in the data series for 1994, 1999, and 2002 due to revised methodologies for determining SNAP eligibility (U.S. Department of Agriculture, 2011b, table 2 and appendix D).

Although SNAP participation decreased by an average 4.6 percent (1.0 million participants) per year over the 1993-2000 period of economic growth (fig. 5), the change in caseload varied markedly over this period. During the first 2 years of economic growth (1993 and 1994), participation increased by an average 4.0 percent (1.0 million participants) per year (appendix B, table 1). The increased participation was probably, in part, the result of the 1993 Omnibus Budget Reconciliation Act (P.L. 103-66) that eased eligibility rules and increased the take-up rate among those eligible.[9,10] A lag in the economic gains to low-income households during the initial period of an economic recovery could have also contributed to the increase in participation (see box, "Asymmetrical Lags in SNAP Participation," p. 11).

Participation finally started to fall in 1995, and the decrease accelerated in 1997 through 2000 following welfare reform and greater State use of short certification periods and frequent recertification (e.g., every 3 months).

The Personal Responsibility and Work Opportunity Reconciliation Act of 1996 (P.L. 104-193, also known as welfare reform), made extensive changes to SNAP that tightened eligibility rules and reduced benefits—changes expected to reduce participation.[11] Welfare reform also made changes to other programs assisting low-income households that discouraged SNAP-eligible households from participating in the program, as reflected in the reduction of the SNAP take-up rate (U.S. Government Accountability Office, 1999; Zedlewski and Gruber, 2001; and U.S. Department of Agriculture, 2001).[12]

While participation fell an average 3.6 percent (1.0 million participants) per year during 1995 to 1996, it fell an average 9.4 percent (2.1 million participants) per year from 1997 to 2000 (appendix B, table 1). Welfare reform augmented the decline in participation that was occurring as a result of economic growth, as reflected in a greater per year reduction in participa- tion during 1997 to 2000, compared with 1995 to 1996. A number of studies (discussed in appendix A) substantiate the impact of welfare reform on SNAP participation, both the legislated changes to SNAP and the cross-program effects of changes in other programs (Currie and Grogger, 2001; Kornfeld, 2002; Kabbani and Wilde, 2003; and Klerman and Danielson, 2011).

The 2001-03 period of economic decline saw participation increase by an average of 7.4 percent (1.4 million participants) per year (fig. 5). Changes to policy and administrative practices boosted the increase in participation that was due to an increase in the unemployment rate. During this time, there was particular concern about the low take-up rates among eligible families with earnings (McKernan and Ratcliffe, 2003; U.S. Government Accountability Office, 2004). A number of efforts were made to turn the falling take-up rate around. Program outreach was expanded, simplified reporting for house- holds with earnings was introduced, transitional benefits for TANF leavers were started, less restrictive State TANF rules for treating a vehicle as an asset could be used instead of SNAP vehicle and asset rules, and expanded categorical eligibility was started (U.S. Government Accountability Office, 2002; Trippe et al., 2004; Zedlewski et al., 2004 and 2005).[13] In response to the changes in policy, the take-up rate started to rise in 2002, adding to the increase in participation resulting from the economic decline (see, Ratcliff, et al., 2008; Mabli, et al., 2009; and Klerman and Danielson, 2011).

Although 2004-07 was a period of economic growth, SNAP participation increased—by an average 5.6 percent (1.3 million participants) per year (fig. 5). Several factors underlie this seemingly contrary result (Ratcliffe, 2008; Mabli et al., 2009; Klerman and Danielson, 2011). First, the take-up rate for eligible households rose during this period, likely a response to continued outreach efforts and adoption of other administrative practices that made enrolling and staying in the program easier, such as streamlining the application process, simplifying the reporting of changes to income while enrolled in the program, and instituting longer certification periods. Second, more States adopted options for using categorical eligibility that likely increased participation. These program changes occurred through the Agriculture Appropriations Act of 2001, USDA-FNS regulations, and the Farm Security and Rural Investment Act of 2002 (P.L. 107-171, 2002 Farm Bill) that also restored eligibility for all legal immigrant children. Third, labor market conditions for less skilled workers, such as real wages and job opportunities, did not improve as much or as quickly as they had during past economic recoveries, and poverty rates remained close to those of the previous period of economic decline (Bivens and Irons, 2008; Blank, 2009; Greenstone and Looney, 2011). Consequently, economic growth as measured by a decrease in the unemployment rate did not alleviate the need for nutri- tion assistance by low-income households.[14] And fourth, a series of hurri- canes in the fall of 2005, including Hurricane Katrina, devastated areas along the Gulf Coast, resulting in a large but mostly temporary increase in partici- pation (Hanson and Oliveira, 2007).

The 2008-10 period of economic decline saw SNAP participation increase by an average 15.4 percent (4.7 million participants) per year (fig. 5). The large increase in participation can be attributable to the economic decline, while the continued use of State policy options and enactment of the American Recovery and Reinvestment Act of 2009 (ARRA, P.L. 111-5) that took effect in April 2009 (USDA, 2010a) could have also contributed to the increase. ARRA, also known as the Stimulus Act, raised the maximum SNAP benefit amount by 13.6 percent, which likely increased the take-up rate among eligible persons (Nord and Prell, 2011).

ARRA also suspended time-limited benefits for able-bodied adults without dependents (ABAWDs) through fiscal 2010, thereby expanding SNAP eligibility. After normalizing to account for the large change in the unemploy- ment rate that occurred during 2008-10, the authors found that SNAP participation increased by an annual average 2.7 million participants per 1-percentage-point increase in the unemployment rate (appendix B, table 6). This was in the range of 2 to 3 million participants per 1-percentage-point increase in the unemployment rate that occurred during the previous two periods of economic decline and during the first half of the 1980-83 period of economic decline. In all these periods, changes in program policy augmented the increase in participation that would have occurred during an economic decline. During the last 2 years of the 1980-83 period, changes in program policy countered the effects of the economic decline and led to a reduction in participation.[15] Only during the 1993-2000 period of economic growth was the annual average decrease of 2.4 million participants per 1-percentage-point decline in the unemployment rate within the 2 to 3 million range of decreases that occurred during the periods of economic decline. Changes in program policy would have augmented the decrease in participation during this period of economic growth. During the other periods of growth, the change in partici- pation per 1-percentage-point decrease in the unemployment rate was either small or it increased due to changes in program policy and other factors that tended to favor participation, countering the tendency for participation to fall with the unemployment rate.

SNAP SUMMARY

The relationship between change in the unemployment rate and SNAP partic- ipation was consistent with expectations of their rising or falling together during six of the eight periods of economic growth and decline in this study (fig. 5). In all four periods of economic decline, participation increased with the unemployment rate as expected, and the magnitude of increase was augmented by changes in program policy in all four periods. After normalizing for the change in the unemployment rate, the authors found the increase in SNAP participation during the 2008-10 period of economic decline to be consistent with the increase during previous periods of economic decline.

In two of the four periods of economic growth (1984-89 and 1993-2000), participation decreased, but in the other two it increased, contrary to expectations.

However, these contrary results for the 1976-79 and 2004-07 growth periods were likely due to changes in program policy that increased participation and to other factors that led to an increase in the poverty rate, such as stagnant real earnings and job opportunities for low-skilled workers, which would have contributed to an increase in participation.

Special Supplemental Nutrition Program for Women, Infants, and Children (WIC)

Initiated as a 2-year pilot program in 1972, WIC officially started in fiscal year 1974. The program's mission is to safeguard the health of low-income pregnant, breastfeeding, and postpartum women, infants, and children up to age 5 who are at nutritional risk by providing supplemental foods, nutrition education, breastfeeding promotion and support, and health care referrals. To be eligible for WIC, applicants must meet income guidelines, a State residency requirement, and be individually determined to be at "nutrition risk" by a health professional. To be eligible on the basis of income, applicants' gross income (before taxes) must fall at or below 185 percent of the U.S. Poverty Income Guidelines. A person who participates or has family members who participate in certain other benefit programs, such as SNAP, Medicaid, or TANF, automatically meets the income eligibility requirement. The amount of food provided to WIC participants does not vary with household income.

For much of the WIC program's history, WIC caseloads were unresponsive to economic conditions. However, evidence suggests that the program has become more responsive since the late 1990s. For example, over the 1976-1997 period, the correlation coefficient between year-to-year change in the unemployment rate and year-to-year change in WIC participation was -

0.16—indicating that there was a small reduction in WIC participation when the unemployment rate increased, contrary to what would be expected. However, the correlation coefficient rose to 0.60 over the more recent years of 1998-2010. The dramatic difference in the relationship between WIC participation and the unemployment rate in these two time periods was due to changes in the program's funding levels. Unlike SNAP, WIC is a discretionary program funded by appropriations law. The number of eligible applicants who can be served depends on the annual appropriation, cost of the foods provided to participants, and other costs of operating the program. When funds are limited, WIC agencies use a priority system to ration benefits to those at the highest nutritional risk. Until the late 1990s, WIC was not fully funded–that is, appropriated funds were not sufficient to serve all eligible applicants who wanted to participate. Since data were not collected on whether applicants were turned away from local WIC clinics because of lack of funds, it is not possible to determine when the program became fully funded. However, anecdotal evidence suggests that sometime in the late 1990s WIC became fully funded, enabling all eligible applicants to the program to participate and making caseloads more responsive to economic conditions. We chose 1998 as the start of the full-funding period. After this time, WIC caseloads appear to have become more responsive to economic conditions. During the pre-full-funding period (1976-97), participation increased each year, regardless of whether the unemployment rate was increasing or decreasing (fig. 6). The rising caseload was due to annual increases in Congressional appropriations that were stimulated largely by evaluations showing WIC to be a successful and cost-effective program.[16] The finding by Bitler, et al. (2003, p. 1,168) that "WIC participation was not strongly related to state-level indicators of need as measured by the unemployment rate and poverty rate," based on data for 1992 to 2000, supports this report's finding that WIC was not sensitive to economic conditions during this pre-full- funding period.

The increase in participation varied during the pre-full-funding period. During 1976-89, participation increased by an average 270,000 participants per year, while during 1990-97 it increased by an average 411,000 partici- pants per year (fig. 7 and appendix B, table 2).[17] The more rapid growth in the annual average number of participants during 1990-97 was due largely to the startup of State-initiated infant formula rebate programs in the late 1980s.[18] Typically, State agencies obtain significant discounts in the form of rebates from infant formula manufacturers for each can of formula purchased through the program, and, in exchange, a manufacturer is given the exclusive right to provide its product to WIC participants in that State. The effect of rebates on costs is substantial. For example, the average cost of the monthly WIC food package in 1998 was $47.03 before rebates and $31.76 after rebates (Bartlett et al., 2000). By lowering costs, the rebate program enabled more eligible persons to be served. The program was so successful that, since 1989, Federal law has required that WIC State agencies enter into cost-containment contracts for the purchase of infant formula used in WIC.

Participation patterns during the pre-full-funding period varied among participant categories. For much of the time, the number of women and infants participating in WIC increased more than the number of children in the program.[19] In general, infants and pregnant and breastfeeding women have a higher priority for participating in WIC than do children, and so they are more likely to be selected to participate when program funds are limited. However, during 1993-97, the number of children participating in the program increased more than infants and women (fig. 7). As program funding expanded and approached full-funding levels, a greater number of lower priority applicants, such as children, were able to participate. At the same time, the number of births declined, which would have reduced the pool of eligible women and infants and thus limited the growth in their participa- tion (for trends in the number of births, see Hamilton et al. (2010) and Sutton and Hamilton (2011)).

Once WIC reached full-funding levels, participation appears to have become more sensitive to the unemployment rate. For instance, during 1998-2000, the economy was expanding and the number of participants fell each year, the only decrease in total participation during the study period (fig. 6). This result is not surprising given that once the program reached full-funding levels, favorable economic conditions would be expected to decrease the number of income-eligible applicants. The reduction in participation occurred through a reduction in the number of children participating in the program (fig. 7). Mothers with children are presumably more able to take advantage of increased employment opportunities resulting from economic growth than are pregnant women and women with infants, thereby reducing the number of children who are income-eligible to participate. Also, a decrease in births during the previous 5 years likely contributed to a decrease in the number of participating children.

Finally, passage of the 1998 William F. Goodling Child Nutrition Reauthorization Act (P.L. 105-336) likely contributed to the decrease in participants by requiring that most WIC applicants be physically present at certification, document their income, and present proof of residency.

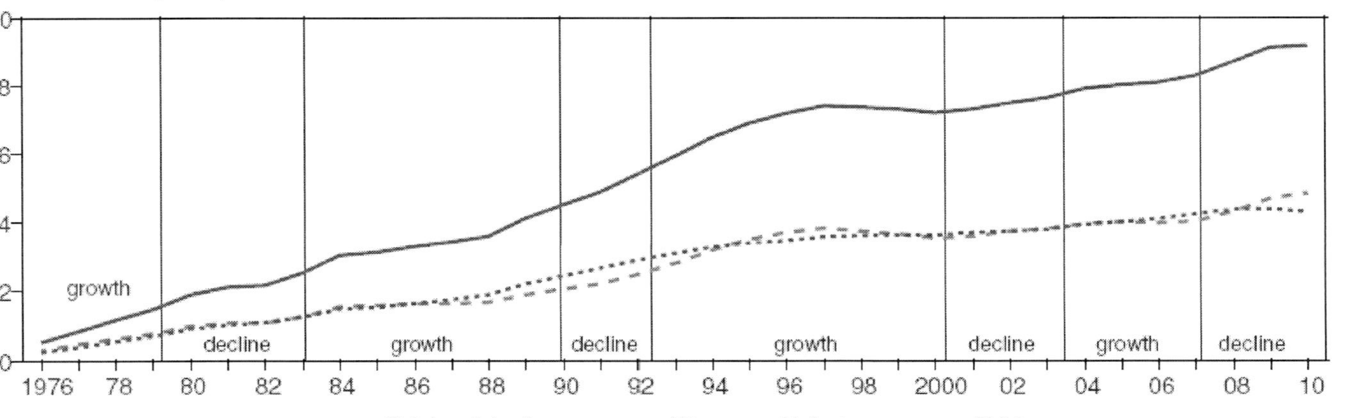

Source: USDA Food and Nutrition Service data.

Figure 6. Special Supplemental Nutrition Program for Women, Infants, and Children (WIC) participation, fiscal years 1976-2010.

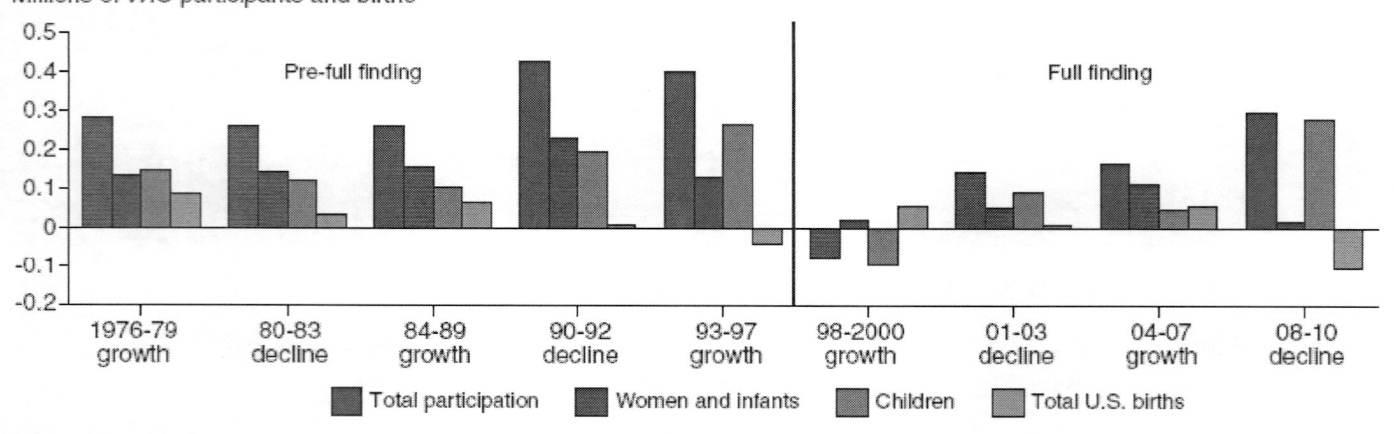

Years shown are fiscal years.

Source: USDA Economic Research Service calculations based on USDA Food and Nutrition Service data and U.S. Department of Health and Human Services data.

Figure 7. Special Supplemental Nutrition Program for Women, Infants, and Children (WIC) participation and births, annual average change during periods of economic growth and decline.

Although total participation and the number of children in WIC fell each year during the 1998-2000 period of economic growth, the number of women and infants in WIC increased slightly (fig. 7); again, pregnant women and women with infants are less likely to be able to take advantage of employment oppor- tunities resulting from economic growth and more likely to meet the WIC income-eligibility requirements.[20] The increase in births during the period also likely contributed to the increase of women and infants in the program.

During the 2001-03 period of economic decline, participation increased by an average 2 percent (146,000 participants) per year (fig. 7). Although there was little change in the number of births during the period, the increase in births during the 1998-2000 period likely contributed to the increase in participa- tion among children during the 2001-03 period.

During the 2004-07 period of economic growth, participation continued to expand by an average 2 percent (164,000 participants) per year. This contrary result was also found in the relationship between SNAP participation and the unemployment rate. Although the economy was growing and the unemploy- ment rate was falling, the poverty rate remained close to the levels reached during the 2001 recession, which suggests that the economic situation for a significant segment of the U.S. population did not improve. It is also likely that the increase in births during the period contributed to this increase in WIC participation.

During the 2008-10 period of rising unemployment, participation increased by an average 3.5 percent (296,000 participants) per year. This increase occurred primarily among children, whose participation increased by an average 6.5 percent (279,000 children) per year (fig. 7). The increase in WIC participation might have been greater during the 2008-10 period, but a decrease in the number of births during these years likely limited the increase in the number of women and infants participating in the program, as well as the number of children.

The increase was larger during the first 2 years of the 2008-10 period, when WIC experienced an average 5 percent (418,000 participants) per year growth in participation—primarily among children, whose number increased by an average 8.2 percent (344,000 children) per year (appendix B, table 2). Despite the continued rise in unemployment in 2010, the growth in WIC participation slowed. For the first time in the program's history, the combined number of women and infants fell, the likely result of a decrease in births during 2010. The number of children in the program continued to increase, but by less than half of the increase during 2008-09. The lower number of births in the previous 2 years may have limited growth in the number of children partici- pating in 2010.[21]

After normalizing for the change in the unemployment rate, the authors found that WIC participation increased by an annual average of 170,000 participants per 1-percentage-point increase in the unemployment rate during the 2008-10 period (appendix B, table 7). Due to the effect of a reduction in births, the increase in participation during this period was somewhat less than the 200,000- to 223,000 change in the number of participants per 1-percentage-point change in the unemployment rate that occurred during two of the other three fully funded periods, 1998-2000 and 2001-03. During the 2004-07 period of economic growth, participation increased despite the fall in the unemployment rate.

WIC Summary

During the pre-full-funding era of WIC, the annual average increase in total participation was budget-driven, and the magnitude of the increase was 50 percent greater when infant formula rebates were implemented in 1989. Since the late 1990s, when the program became fully funded, partici- pation appears to have responded to the unemployment rate, although the relationship between the unemployment rate and WIC participation was also influenced by the number of births. After full funding, WIC participa- tion increased during the two periods of economic decline that followed (2001-03 and 2008-10) and decreased during one of the two periods of economic growth (1998-2000). During the other period of economic growth (2004-07), WIC participation increased as poverty rates remained high despite a declining unemployment rate (a similar pattern was observed with SNAP participation).

Changes in the number of births affected the magnitude of changes in participation, as during 2008-10, when a reduc- tion in the number of births led to a decrease in participation by women and infants in 2010 and only a small increase during 2008-09, limiting the growth in participation that would normally have occurred in response to the economic decline. These results point out the importance of taking the trend in births into account in analyzing the relationship between WIC participation and the unemployment rate.

National School Lunch Program (NSLP)

Established in 1946, NSLP—the largest of USDA's child nutrition programs— provides nutritious lunches at low or no cost to students. Schools that choose to participate in the program receive cash subsidies and foods from USDA to offset the cost of food service. In return, the schools must serve lunches that meet Federal nutrition requirements and offer free or reduced-price lunches to needy children. Any student in attendance at a participating school is entitled to participate in the program. Children from families with incomes at or below 130 percent of the Federal poverty guidelines are eligible for free meals, and those from families with incomes greater than 130 percent and at or below 185 percent of the poverty guidelines are eligible for reduced-price meals. Children from families with incomes over 185 percent of the poverty guidelines pay full price, although their meals are still subsidized to a small extent. In 2010, 90 percent of U.S. students were in schools, both public and private, that chose to offer the program. That same year, 57 percent of all students participated in the NSLP, with 55 percent of them receiving free meals, 10 percent receiving reduced-price meals, and 35 percent receiving full-price meals.

Economic conditions do not appear to have any impact on the total number of students receiving school lunches (see box, "National School Lunch Program (NSLP) Total Participation and the Unemployment Rate," p. 22). However, there is evidence that the economy does affect the percentage of NSLP partici-pants receiving free and reduced-price meals (fig. 8).[22] As economic conditions decline, household income falls, and more participants become eligible for free and reduced-price meals. Consequently the percentage of NSLP participants receiving free and reduced-price meals tends to increase. Because the number of participants receiving free and reduced-price meals also increased during each year of the study with the growth in school enrollment, the percentage receiving free and reduced-price meals is a better indicator for measuring the influence of economic conditions than the number of participants.

During the 1976-79 growth period, the percentage of NSLP participants receiving free and reduced-price meals increased an average 2 percent per year, contrary to expectations (fig. 9 and appendix B, table 3).[23] However, the percentage of NSLP participants receiving free and reduced-price meals increased during the first 2 years and decreased during the last 2 years of the period. The favorable economic conditions during the period likely contrib-uted to the reduction in the percentage of NSLP participants receiving free and reduced-price meals that occurred during 1978-79, the first decrease since implementation of the free and reduced-price meal system (fig. 8). The increase during 1976-77 was the continuation of a past trend, reflecting an increase in program availability during an era of program expansion.

The percentage of NSLP participants receiving free and reduced-price meals increased during 1980-83 by an average 4.3 percent per year (fig. 9). However, this result was not due to a shift in participation from full-price to free and reduced-price meals, but rather to a large reduction (average 7.4 percent per year) in full-price participants due to program policy changes along with only a small (average 0.4 percent per year) increase in free and reduced-price participation. The Omnibus Budget Reconciliation Act of 1981 reduced the Federal reimbursement rates paid to schools for both full-price and reduced-price lunches. As a result of the decreased reimbursement, some schools dropped out of the program. In addition, some of the schools that remained in the program responded by raising the prices of school meals, and some students reacted by bringing their lunches rather than paying the higher prices (U.S. General Accounting Office, 1984), reducing the number of participants receiving full-price meals.[24]

During the 1984-89 period of economic growth, the percentage of NSLP participants receiving free and reduced-price meals decreased by an average 1.6 percent per year (fig. 9). This was the only period in which the percent of participants receiving free and reduced-price meals decreased. During the 1990-92 period of economic decline, the percentage of NSLP participants receiving free and reduced-price meals increased by an average 4 percent per year (fig. 9). This resulted from an increase in the number of participants receiving free and reduced-price meals by an average 4.6 percent (540,000) per year and a decrease in the number of participants receiving full-price meals by an average 3.2 percent (400,000) per year (fig. 10 and appendix B, table 3). This shift from full-price meals to free and reduced-price meals is what would be expected during an economic decline.

Direct certification, implemented during the 1990-92 period, likely augmented the increase in the percentage of participants receiving free and reduced-price meals due to economic conditions. Prior to the 1990s, all families who wanted their children to receive free or reduced-price meals had to complete and submit application forms to their school; the schools then applied eligibility rules to determine whether the children qualified.

In 1989, Public Law 101-147 (the Child Nutrition and WIC Reauthorization Act of 1989) granted school food authorities the option to certify children for free school meals with direct certification by using documentation from the

State or local welfare office indicating that a child was a member of a household receiving food stamps or benefits from AFDC (U.S. Department of Agriculture, 2010b). A study of the direct certification process by Jackson et al. (2000) found that school districts began using direct certification in 1991, and by fall 1996, it was being used in 63 percent of all NSLP districts, representing 72 percent of all students nationwide. Jackson et al. estimated "that each additional year of direct certification leads to a statistically significant increase of 0.27 percentage points in the percent of enrollment that participates in the lunch program and receives free meals."

National School Lunch Program (NSLP) Total Participation and the Unemployment Rate

Unlike SNAP and WIC programs, in which receipt of benefits is tied to income, all children attending schools that offer NSLP may participate regardless of their family's income. While NSLP is available to the vast majority of schoolchildren, close to 40 percent do not participate in the program. The question is whether nonparticipating students, most of whom are probably above the income cutoff level for free and reduced-price meals, would be influenced to participate as economic conditions decline. For example, some parents who prepare a lunch for their children or give them money to eat off-campus may save by having the children get a school meal, even at full price (though subsidized to some extent). Other parents of children participating in the program at full price may decide they can economize by packing an inexpensive meal prepared at home. The point is that changes in economic conditions could affect the participation decisions not just of those eligible for free and reduced- price meals, but also of those who must pay for a full-price meal. However, the data suggest that the number of children participating in the NSLP bears little relationship to economic conditions (fig. 8). In fact, the correlation coefficient between the year-to-year change in NSLP participants and the year-to- year change in the unemployment rate from 1976 to 2010 was -0.35; the negative value means that a rise in the unemployment rate is actually associated with a decrease in NSLP participation. Throughout most of the study period, the number of NSLP participants increased each year regardless of whether the economy was growing or in decline.[1] The percent of students who participated in the program was stable over the study period, with an average of 53 percent, a maximum of 58 percent, and a minimum of 50 percent.

Consequently, total participation in the NSLP does not appear to be affected by economic conditions. Instead, it is closely related to school enrollment, with a correlation coefficient of 0.88 during the study period (fig. 8).

[1] The only exception was a 3-year period from 1980 through 1982 that coincided with a falling school enrollment and the enactment of the Omnibus Budget Reconciliation Act of 1981 (P.L. 97-35), which tightened the eligibility criteria for both schools and students and decreased the Federal reimbursement rates for school meals (U.S. General Account- ing Office, 1984).

During the economic growth period 1993-2000, the percentage of NSLP partic- ipants receiving free and reduced-price meals continued to increase, although by an average of only 1 percent per year (fig. 9). Some of this contrary result may be explained by the continued implementation of direct certification. But by the late 1990s, the adoption of direct certification had slowed (Jackson et al., 2000) and the percentage of NSLP participants receiving free and reduced-price meals started to fall (fig. 8). This decrease was reinforced when the Personal Responsibility and Work Opportunity Reconciliation Act of 1996 (P.L. 104-193, also known as welfare reform), replaced the AFDC program with the TANF program. Because fewer children were eligible for TANF than had been eligible under AFDC, fewer were now eligible for free school meals under direct certification (Jackson et al., 2000).

As expected, the percentage of NSLP students receiving free and reduced-price meals increased during the 2001-03 period of economic decline. However, the average 0.8 percent increase per year in the percentage of free and reduced-price meals was smaller than in all other periods of economic decline (fig. 9).

Counter to expectations regarding the effect of economic conditions, the percentage of free and reduced-price meals continued to increase during the 2004-07 economic growth period, although at the low average rate of 0.4 percent per year.

Once again, policy changes related to direct certifica- tion may have played a role in the increase in participation during a period of economic growth. In an effort to enroll more eligible children for free meals in the NSLP, the Child Nutrition and WIC Reauthorization Act of 2004 (Public Law 108-265) required all school districts to establish a system of direct certification of children from households participating in SNAP. Until then, direct certification was still optional for school districts (U.S. Department of Agriculture, 2010b).

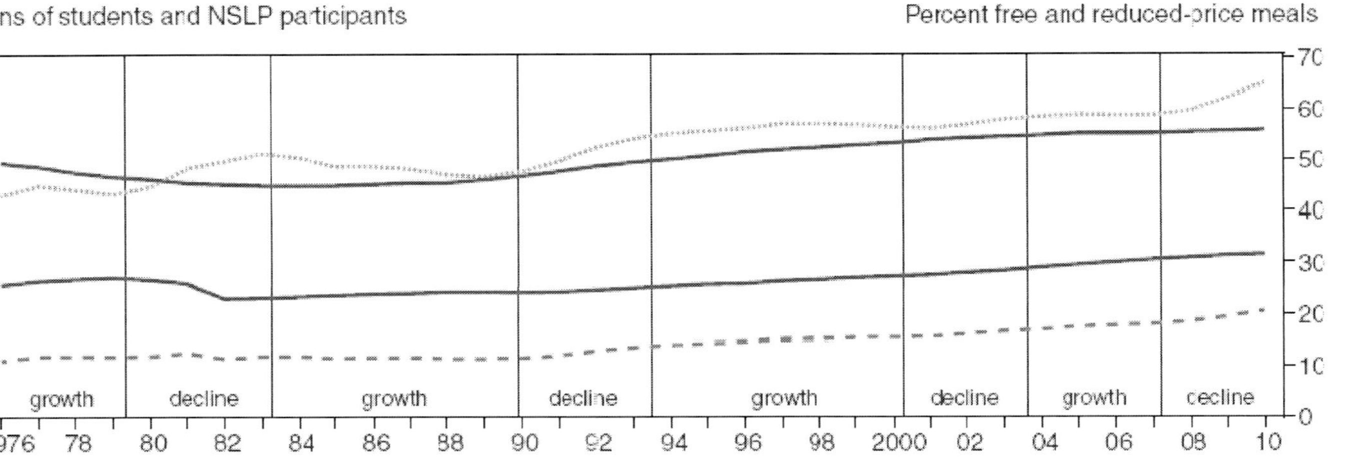

Source: USDA Food and Nutrition Service data and U.S. Department of Education data.

Figure 8. National School Lunch Program (NSLP) participation, school enrollment, and percentage of participants receiving free and reduced-price meals, fiscal years 1976-2010.

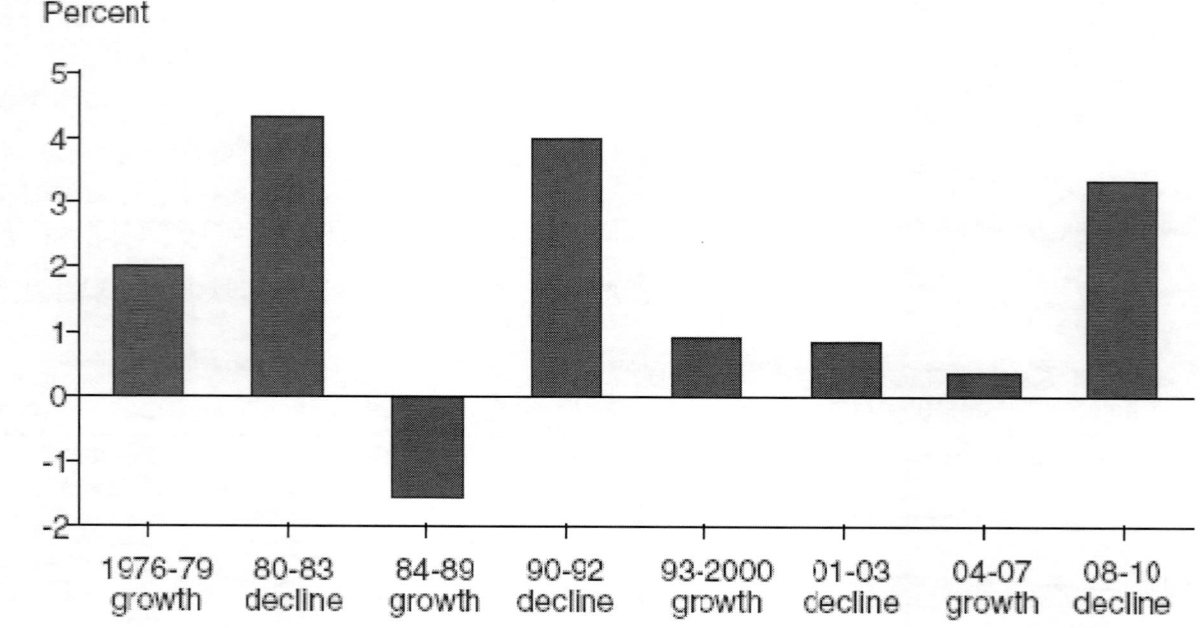

Source: USDA Economic Research Service, based on USDA Food and Nutrition Service data.

Figure 9. Annual average percent change in percentage of National School Lunch Program (NSLP) participants receiving free and reduced-price meals during periods of economic growth (blue) and decline (red).

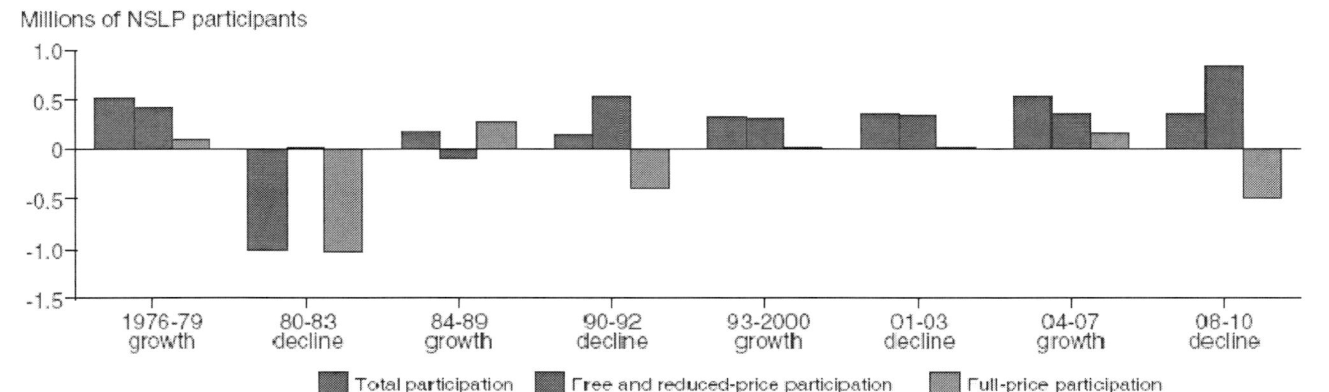

Source: USDA Economic Research Service calculations based on USDA Food and Nutrition Service data.

Figure 10. National School Lunch Program (NSLP) participation: annual average change during periods of economic growth and decline.

The mandate was to be phased in over 3 years: the largest local educational agencies were required to establish direct certification systems by school year 2006-07, and all local educational agen- cies were required to directly certify SNAP participants by school year 2008-09. However, many State agencies—recognizing that direct certification, would increase participation, ease the burden on families and local educa- tional agencies, and result in more accurate targeting of free school meal benefits—chose to phase in direct certification in advance of the mandate (U.S. Department of Agriculture, 2010b).

So during a time of economic growth when the percentage of free and reduced-price meals would be expected to decrease, States were expanding their use of direct certification, and the percentage of NSLP participants receiving free and reduced-price meals increased slightly.[25]

During the 2008-10 period of economic decline, the percentage of NSLP participants receiving free and reduced-price meals increased by an annual average 3.3 percent per year (fig. 9), reaching a historical high of 65 percent of participants in 2010 (fig. 8). The rise was a result of an increase in the number of students receiving free or reduced-price meals and a decrease in the number paying full price (fig. 10).

Although the change in the percentage of NSLP participants receiving free and reduced-price meals likely would have occurred even in the absence of direct certification, the legislative mandate in 2004 requiring all school districts to establish such certifica-tion by school year 2008-09 may have contributed to the increase due to the record SNAP caseloads during this period. After normalizing for the change in the unemployment rate, the authors found that the percentage of NSLP participants receiving free and reduced-price meals increased by an annual average of 1.9 percent per 1-percentage-point increase in the unemployment rate during the 2008-10 period (appendix B, table 8). The 1.9-percent change falls into the lower end of the 1.3 to 5.5 percent range that occurred during the three other periods of economic decline.

The two highest increases were likely influenced by changes to program policy: direct certification during the 1990-92 period and the budget reconciliation acts during the 1980-83 period. Only in the 1984-89 period of economic growth was the annual average 1.9-percent decrease within the range that the percentage of free and reduced-price meals increased during the periods of economic decline.

NSLP Summary

Economic conditions tend to influence the percentage of NSLP participants receiving free and reduced-price meals but not the total number of NSLP participants.

During the last three periods of economic decline, the percentage of students participating in the NSLP who received free or reduced-price meals increased by an average 1 to 4 percent per year. Only during the 1983-89 period of economic growth did the percentage of students receiving free and reduced-price meals fall as expected.

Although during the other periods of growth the percentage increased contrary to expecta- tions, the increase was small relative to the increase during periods of economic decline. Direct certification was one policy that tended to increase the percentage of participants receiving free and reduced-price meals, even during periods of economic growth.

School Breakfast Program (SBP)

Established in 1966 as a pilot program, the SBP was made permanent in 1975. The program provides nutritious breakfasts at low or no cost to students. Schools that choose to participate in the program receive cash subsidies from USDA to offset the cost of food service. In return, the schools must serve break- fasts that meet Federal nutrition requirements and offer free or reduced-price breakfasts to needy children. Unlike NSLP, schools may qualify for higher "severe need" reimbursements if 40 percent of their lunches for the prior 2 years were served free or at a reduced price. Any student attending a partici- pating school is entitled to participate in the program. Children from families with incomes at or below 130 percent of the Federal poverty guidelines are eligible for free meals, and those from families with incomes greater than 130 percent and at or below 185 percent of the poverty guidelines are eligible for reduced-price meals. Children from families with incomes over 185 percent of the poverty guidelines pay full price, although their meals are still subsidized to a small extent. In 2010, 81 percent of students were in schools, both public and private, that chose to participate in the program. That same year, 21 percent of student enrollment participated in the SBP, with 74 percent of SBP participants receiving free meals, 9 percent receiving reduced-price meals, and 17 percent paying full price.

As with the NSLP, economic conditions do not appear to have any impact on the total number of students receiving school breakfasts (see box, "School Breakfast Program (SBP) Total Participation and the Unemployment Rate," p. 28).

There is evidence, however, that the economy does impact the percentage of SBP participants receiving free and reduced-price meals (fig. 11). The percentage of SBP participants receiving free and reduced-price meals increased an average 0.6 percent per year during the 1976-79 period of economic growth (fig. 12 and appendix B, table 4).

Although this result was contrary to expectations, the favorable economic conditions apparently had an impact during the latter half of this period as the percentage of SBP partici- pants receiving free and reduced-price meals decreased in both 1978 and 1979.

During the first several years after the program was permanently authorized, it was targeted to schools in low-income areas with a greater need for subsi- dized breakfasts, and thus there was an increase in the percentage of free and reduced-price meals.

The percentage of SBP participants receiving free and reduced-price meals increased by an average 1.8 percent per year during the 1980-83 period of economic decline, the largest average annual change for the program among the eight economic periods (fig. 12).

As with the NSLP, however, the increase was probably due as much to the Omnibus Budget Reconciliation Act of 1981 as to economic conditions.[26]

As expected, the percentage of SBP participants receiving free and reduced-price meals decreased by an average 0.6 percent per year during the 1984-89 period of economic growth, increased by an average 0.4 percent per year during the 1990-92 period of decline, and then decreased by an average 0.5 percent per year during the 1993-2000 period of economic growth (fig. 12).

It is possible that grants to schools to help start up the SBP, which were reauthorized in 1994 legislation (extending 1989 legislation), influenced the decrease in the percentage of SBP participants receiving free and reduced-price meals during the 1993-2000 period of growth.

As program availability expanded into higher income areas, it was likely that the percentage of participants receiving free and reduced-price meals would decrease as schools with a greater need for subsi- dized breakfasts would already have entered the program.

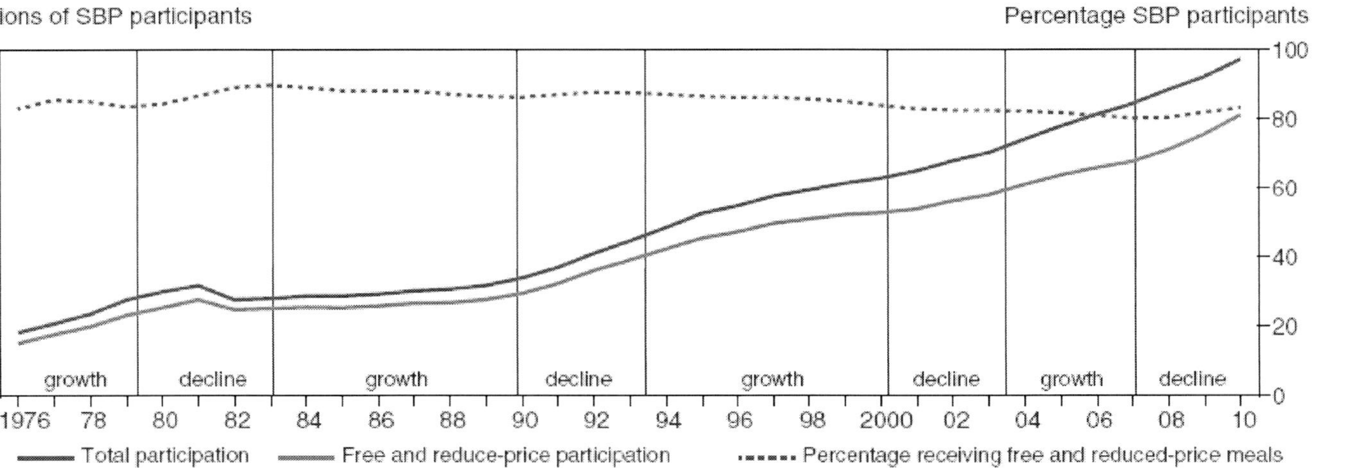

Source: USDA Food and Nutrition Service data.

Figure 11. School Breakfast Program (SBP) participation and percentage of participants receiving free and reduced-price meals, fiscal years 1976-2010.

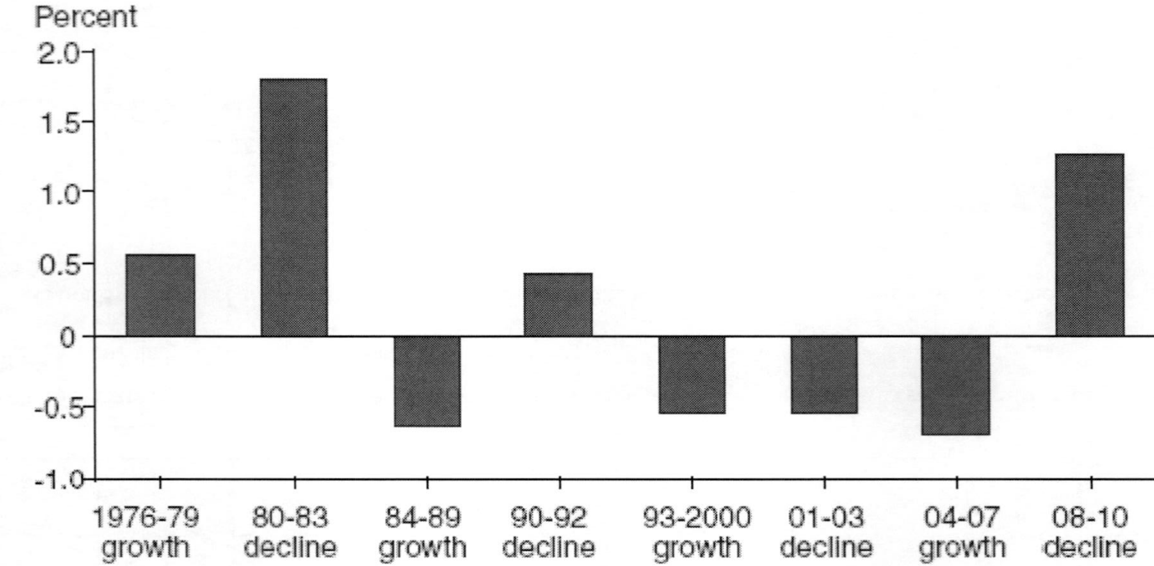

Source: USDA Economic Research Service, based on USDA Food and Nutrition Service data.

Figure 12. Annual average percent change in percentage of School Breakfast Program (SBP) participants receiving free and reduced-price meals during periods of economic growth (blue) and decline (red).

School Breakfast Program (SBP) Total Participation and the Unemployment Rate

The number of SBP participants is largely determined by school enrollment and the decision by schools to make the program available to students, with economic conditions playing a minor role, if any. The correlation coefficient between the year-to- year change in SBP participation and the year-to-year change in the unemployment rate from 1976 to 2010, the period of the study, was very small at 0.03. Over almost the entire period, participation in the program increased each year, regardless of whether the economy was growing or in decline (fig. 11).[1] After growing slowly in the 1980s, participation increased at a faster rate starting around 1990, which coincided with the passage of the Child Nutrition and WIC Reauthorization Act of 1989 that provided special grants to States to help defray the costs of starting up new School Breakfast Programs (P.L. 101-147).[2]

From 1990 to 2010, participation in the SBP increased at a rate of 5.5 percent per year (fig. 11). This was over four times greater than the annual average 1.3 percent increase in total National School Lunch Program (NSLP) participation over the same period and over five times greater than the annual average 0.9 percent increase in school enrollment. The fact that the SBP is a relatively young program (it was not granted permanent authorization until 1975) helps explain why it grew much faster than the NSLP during the study period. The availability of the program—that is, the percent of all students enrolled in schools that offer the school meals—started out significantly lower for SBP than for NSLP, which has been widely available since the 1970s (box fig.). For example, in 1976, over 90 percent of students attended a school that participated in the NSLP, compared with less than 20 percent of students who attended a school participating in the SBP. As more schools joined the SBP, program availability approached that of the NSLP, which remained basically unchanged. By 2010, 81 percent of all students attended a school that participated in the SBP, compared with 90 percent who attended a school participating in the NSLP. Despite its relatively faster growth, the average number of participants in the SBP is only about 36 percent that of the NSLP. Although program availability rates between the two programs have converged, student participation rates—the percentage of students in schools that offer NSLP or SBP who receive school meals—differ widely. From 1983 to 2010, the average participation rate for the NSLP was 59 percent, compared with only 22 percent for the SBP.

There was little change in the participation rate for either program over this period.

1The only exception was in 1982 when the Omnibus Budget Reconciliation Act of 1981 (P.L. 97-35) reduced the Federal reimburse- ment rates to schools for school meals, causing schools to raise the prices of school meals, which led to a drop in participation (see the previous chapter on NSLP for more information on the legislation).

2The legislation authorized funds for the start-up grants through fiscal 1994. The Healthy Meals for Healthy Americans Act of 1994 (P.L. 103-448) made the start-up grants permanent and also expanded coverage to include SBP expansion (U.S. Department of Agriculture, 1996).

Program availability for SBP and NSLP: Percent of students enrolled in schools offering the programs, fiscal years 1976-2010

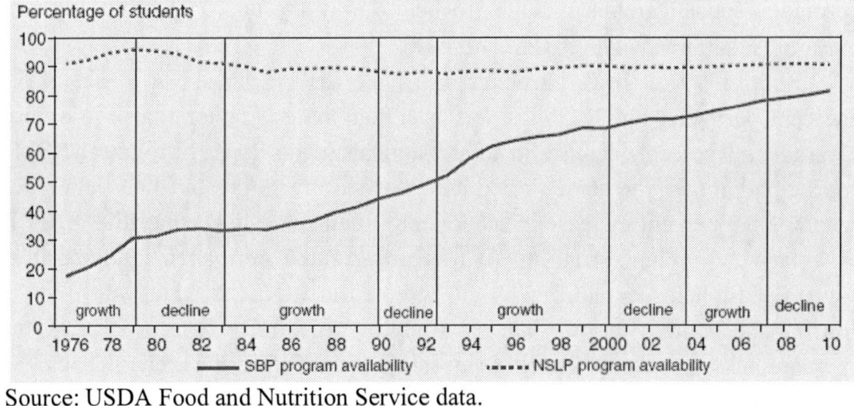

Source: USDA Food and Nutrition Service data.

Counter to expectations, during the 2001-03 period of economic decline the percentage of SBP participants receiving free and reduced-price meals decreased by an average 0.5 percent per year (fig. 12), while—as expected—the percentage of SBP participants receiving free and reduced-price meals decreased by an average 0.7 percent per year during the 2004-07 period of economic growth.

As with earlier periods, it is possible that the continued expansion of program availability would have been in higher income areas with less need for subsidized breakfasts, contributing to the decrease in the percentage of SBP participants receiving free and reduced-price meals during both of these periods.

During the 2008-10 period of economic decline, the percentage of SBP participants receiving free and reduced-price meals increased by an average 1.3 percent per year.

Total participation increased as part of a long-term trend, and the increase in the number of participants who received free and reduced-price meals was about equal to the increase in total participation, while the change in the number of participants paying full price decreased slightly (appendix B, table 4). This shift, though not large, is as expected during a period of economic decline.

After normalizing for the change in the unemployment rate, the authors found that the percentage of SBP participants receiving free and reduced-price meals increased by an annual average 0.7 percent per 1-percentage-point increase in the unemployment rate during the 2008-10 period (appendix B, table 9).

This change was close to the annual average 0.6-percent increase during the 1990-92 period of economic decline, but not at all similar to the change during the other periods of economic decline, a likely outcome of policy changes. In the three most recent periods of economic growth, there was an annual average 0.8- to 1.9-percent decrease in the percentage of SBP participants receiving free and reduced-price meals per 1-percentage-point decrease in the unemployment rate.

SBP Summary

The total number of participants in the SBP does not appear to be related to economic conditions. For almost the entire study period of 1976-2010, participation in the program increased each year—regardless of whether the economy was growing or in decline—as school enrollment and the number of schools offering the program grew. On the other hand, economic conditions do appear to affect the percentage of SBP participants receiving free or reduced-price meals. In three of the four periods of economic decline, the percentage of participants receiving free or reduced-price meals increased, and in three of the four periods of economic growth, that percentage decreased.

The percentage of participants receiving free and reduced-price meals has always been greater in SBP (83 percent in 2010) than in NSLP (65 percent in 2010), and the economy's effect on the percentage of SBP participants receiving free and reduced-price meals—especially during the periods of economic decline—has been much less than its effect on the NSLP.

Child and Adult Care Food Program (CACFP)

Established in 1968, CACFP provides economic incentives for day care facili- ties to provide nutritious meals that contribute to the wellness, healthy growth, and development of young children and the health and wellness of adults in day care. The program reimburses providers for meals served to eligible chil- dren and adults who are enrolled for care at participating day care homes, child care centers, and adult day care centers. CACFP also provides meals and snacks to at-risk children and youth who participate in eligible after- school programs or reside in emergency shelters. Providers of care are reim- bursed at fixed rates per meal, with different reimbursement rates for each type of meal served (breakfast, lunch, dinner, and snack).

In the day care homes portion of CACFP, participating homes (i.e., homes in which the providers care for children other than their own or a combina- tion of others' children and their own children) are reimbursed for meals and snacks at two rates. Homes that are either located in low-income areas or run by a provider whose family income is at or below 185 percent of the Federal poverty guideline receive higher (tier I) rates. Other homes receive lower (tier II) rates, with meals and snacks served to low-income children reimbursed at the tier I rates.

Day care centers are also reimbursed by type of meal served, but at three different rates depending on the family incomes of the children in care. Free and reduced-price eligibility rules and reimbursement rates are identical to those in the NSLP and SBP. Eligible public or private nonprofit child care centers, outside-school-hours care centers, Head Start programs, and other institutions licensed or approved to provide day care services, may participate in CACFP, either independently or as sponsored centers.

Under the program's adult care portion, CACFP provides meals and snacks to adults who receive care in nonresidential adult day care centers. Public or private nonprofit adult day care facilities that provide structured, comprehen- sive services to nonresidential adults who are functionally impaired or aged 60 and older may participate in CACFP as independent or sponsored centers. In 2010, 3.4 million participants received 1,910 million meals. Adults received 3.5 percent of the meals, while the remaining 96.5 percent of the meals were served to children in child care homes (31.2 percent) and in child care centers (65.3 percent). Eighty-two percent of all meals served in the program were free or reduced-price.

As with the other child nutrition programs, economic conditions do not appear to have an impact on the total number of CACFP meals (see box, "Child and Adult Care Food Program (CACFP) Total Participation and the Unemployment Rate," p. 32). However, there is evidence that the economy does impact the percentage of CACFP meals that are free and reduced-price (fig. 13).[27]

In general, when economic conditions declined over the study period (1976-2010), the percentage of total meals that were free and reduced- price increased, and when economic conditions improved, the percentage decreased. Program policy changes also affected the percentage of meals that were free and reduced-price.

Child and Adult Care Food Program (CACFP) Total Participation and the Unemployment

As in the other child nutrition programs examined in this report (NSLP and SBP), overall participation in CACFP does not appear to be related to economic conditions. The correlation coefficient between the year-to-year change in CACFP participation and the year-to-year change in the unemployment rate from 1976 to 2010 was negligible at 0.04. In fact, throughout the entire study period, the number of CACFP participants increased each year regardless of whether the economy was growing or in decline (fig. 13). The number of participants is a function of the availability of the program, which is dependent on the number of centers and sponsoring organizations that choose to participate.[1] The number of these day care centers and sponsoring organizations has increased each year since 1982 (the first year that data were available).

There have been three distinct phases of caseload growth, distinguished by changes in program legislation. The growth in caseloads during these three phases is described in appendix C, Child and Adult Care Food Program (CACFP) Total Participation.

[1]Family child care providers must go through a food sponsor (a public or nonprofit private organization responsible for administration of the program) and cannot apply to the program directly.

During the economic growth period of 1976-79, the percentage of total CACFP meals that were free and reduced-price fell by an average 2.2 percent per year (fig. 14 and appendix B, table 5). Legislation in 1975 (P.L. 94-105) established a three-tiered reimbursement structure that likely reduced the percentage of free and reduced-price meals.

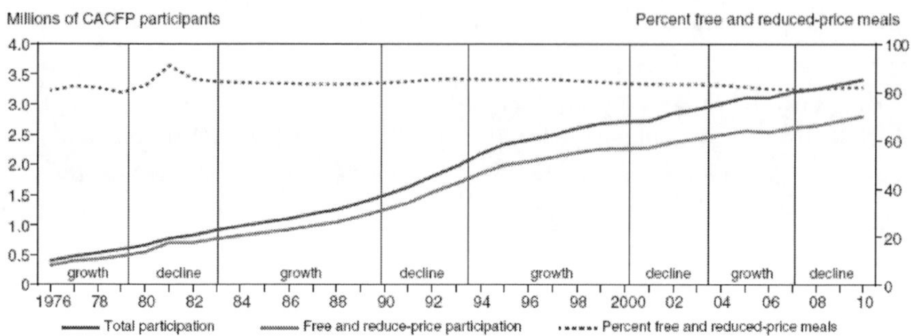

Source: USDA Food and Nutrition Service data.

Figure 13. Child and Adult Care Food Program (CACFP) participation and percentage of total meals that were free and reduced-price, fiscal years 1976-2010.

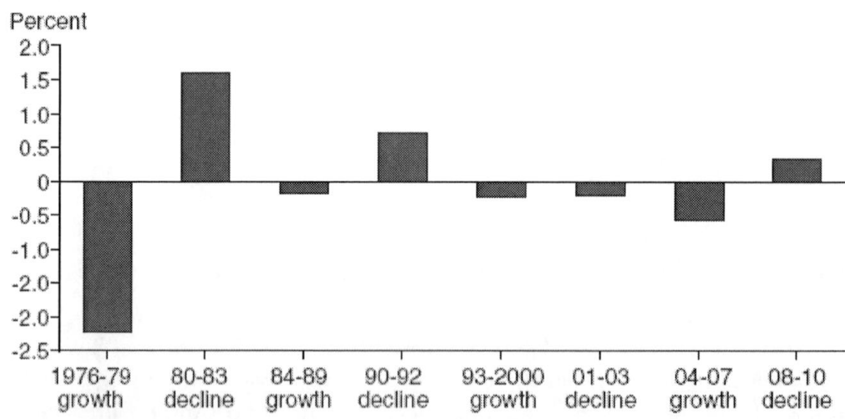

Years shown are fiscal years.

Source: USDA Economic Research Service, based on USDA Food and Nutrition Service data.

Figure 14. Annual average percent change in percentage of total Child and Adult Care Food Program (CACFP) meals that were free and reduced-price meals during periods of economic growth (blue) and decline (red).

During the 1980-83 period of economic decline that followed, the percentage of total meals that were free and reduced-price increased by an average 1.6 percent per year. However, the average over the period obscures the sharp increase over the first half of the period followed by a sharp decrease in the latter half (fig. 13). The change to the reimbursement structure in the 1978 legislation (P.L. 95-627) would have increased the percentage of free and reduced-price meals during 1980 and 1981, while the Omnibus Budget Reconciliation Act of 1981, which reduced reimbursement rates, limited reimbursement to two meals and one snack per child per day, and lowered the eligible age limit to 12, would have decreased the percentage of free and reduced-price meals in 1982 and 1983 (U.S. Department of Agriculture, 2011c).

Subsequent changes in the percentage of meals that were free and reduced-price were small (less than 1 percent) and usually in the expected direction (fig. 14). The percentage decreased by an average of 0.2 percent per year during the 1984-89 period of economic growth, increased by 0.7 percent per year during the 1990-92 period of decline, and decreased by 0.24 percent per year during the 1993-2000 period of economic growth. The relatively larger change during the 1990-92 period may have been influenced by the Child Nutrition and WIC Reauthorization Act of 1989 (P.L. 101-147) that provided funds to expand family day care homes into low-income or rural areas. The enactment of the Personal Responsibility and Work Opportunities Reconciliation Act (PRWORA) in 1996 probably contributed to the decrease in the percentage of free and reduced-price meals during the 1993-2000 period by lowering the maximum number of daily meals and snacks that could be reimbursed in child care centers from four to three and by imple- menting a two-tiered reimbursement structure for day care homes, which tended to decrease the number of day care homes that provided free and reduced-price meals.

The 2001-03 period of economic decline was the only period in which the change in the percentage of CACFP meals that were free and reduced-price was opposite to what would be expected. But the percentage decrease was small, only 0.2 percent per year (fig. 14). The percentage of meals that were free and reduced-price decreased during the economic growth period of 2004-07, as expected, falling by 0.6 percent per year, and increased by 0.3 percent per year during the 2008-10 period of economic decline. During this period of economic decline, the total number of meals served increased as part of a long-term trend, and the increase in the number of meals that were free and reduced-price was about equal to the increase in total meals.

After normalizing for the change in the unemployment rate, the authors found that the percent of total CACFP meals that were free and reduced- price increased by an annual average 0.2 percent per 1-percentage-point increase in the unemployment rate during the 2008-10 period (appendix B, table 10). The change was small and suggests that the percentage of meals served as free and reduced-price is not strongly influenced by a change in economic conditions.

CACFP Summary

Total participation in CACFP shows little relationship to economic conditions. Throughout the history of the program, participation has increased each year regardless of whether the economy was growing or in decline, with the degree of growth influenced by changes in program legisla-tion. However, there is evidence that economic conditions impacted the percentage of CACFP meals that were free and reduced-price. In three of the four periods of economic decline, the percentage of meals that were free or reduced-price increased, and in all four periods of economic growth, the percentage of such meals decreased. However, the year-to-year change was relatively small, as the percentage of CACFP meals that were free or reduced-price ranged between 80 and 85.5 percent during nearly all of the 1976-2010 study period (fig. 13).

Discussion

USDA's nutrition assistance programs are designed to provide nutrition assis- tance to those in need. As economic conditions decline, more people are in need of such assistance. The extent to which the programs respond to economic conditions is one measure of their effectiveness. The results of this study indicate that SNAP, as expected, is the nutrition assistance program that is most responsive to changes in economic conditions, with participation in the program clearly following the unemployment rate—the measure of economic growth or decline used in the study—over the business cycle. However, the study reveals that the other four major nutrition assistance programs are also impacted to some degree by economic conditions. Thus, all of the major nutrition assistance programs are countercyclical, responding to increased demand for their services by needy families during economic downturns.

During the recent 2008-10 period of economic decline, which encompassed the Great Recession, participation in SNAP and WIC and the percentage of participants receiving free and reduced-price meals in all three of the child nutrition programs (NSLP, SBP, and CACFP) increased in response to the rising unemployment rate. For SNAP, the increase in participation during this period was especially large, far exceeding that of the previous three periods of economic decline. The increase in WIC participation also exceeded that of the previous period of economic decline since the program reached full-funding levels in the late 1990s. The increase in the percentage of NSLP and SBP participants receiving free and reduced-price meals was large relative to some previous periods of economic decline. These results are not surprising given the depth of the economic decline during this period of the study, when the largest percentage-point increase in the unemployment rate occurred.

For all programs except CACFP, the changes in participation, normalized for the change in the unemployment rate during the 2008-10 period of economic decline, were generally in line with those of the previous periods of economic decline. The consistency of the participation response among periods of economic decline for these programs, after normalizing, suggests that the large participation response during the 2008-10 period of economic decline reflects the magnitude of the economic downturn during the Great Recession.

Our review of the history of each program reveals that there were many changes to program policies and other factors that affected participation (table 3). Unraveling the effects of the various factors is a challenging task. Previous econometric analyses of the relationship of the unemployment rate and participation in SNAP—the most studied of all the nutrition assistance programs—have been able to explain only about 50 percent of the change in program participation (Klerman and Danielson, 2011; Mabli et al., 2009). Research on participation in the non-SNAP programs that separates the impacts due to economic conditions from those due to policy and other factors is needed to enable policymakers and program analysts to better antic- ipate and forecast fluctuations in participation that can influence budgetary decisions for the programs. Isolating the impacts of the various factors on program participation will also increase our understanding of the effects of policies and help guide future policy decisions.

Table 3. Potential factors affecting participation levels and expected effect, by program, fiscal years 1976-2010

	Periods of economic growth				Periods of economic decline			
Program	1976-79	1984-89	1993-2000	2004-07	1980-83	1990-92	2001-03	2008-10
SNAP								
Unemployment rate	(-)	(-)	(-)	(-)	(+)	(+)	(+)	(+)
Program policy	(+)	(+)	(+/-)	(+)	(+/-)	(+)	(+)	(+)
Natural disasters[1]				(+)				
Other economic factors[2]				(+)				
WIC:[3]								
Unemployment rate			(-)	(-)			(+)	(+)
Program policy			(+/-)			(+)		
Funding levels	(-)	(-)	(-)		(-)	(-)		
Demographics (births)			(+/-)	(+)				(-)
Other economic factors[2]				(+)				
NSLP:								
Program policy					(-)			
Demographics (school enrollment)	(+)	(+)	(+)	(+)	(-)	(+)	(+)	(+)
SBP:								
Program policy					(-)			
Program availability	(+)	(+)	(+)	(+)		(+)	(+)	(+)
Demographics (school enrollment)	(-)	(+)	(+)	(+)	(-)	(+)	(+)	(+)
CACFP:								
Program policy	(+)		(-)			(+)		
Program availability	(+)	(+)	(+)	(+)	(+)	(+)	(+)	(+)

Program	Periods of economic growth				Periods of economic decline			
	1976-79	1984-89	1993-2000	2004-07	1980-83	1990-92	2001-03	2008-10
Potential factors affecting percent of participants receiving free and reduced price meals and expected effect, by program								
NSLP:								
Unemployment rate	(-)	(-)	(-)	(-)	(+)	(+)	(+)	(+)
Program policy			(+/-)	(+)	(+)	(+)		
Other economic factors[2]				(+)				
SBP:								
Unemployment rate	(-)	(-)	(-)	(-)	(+)	(+)	(+)	(+)
Program policy	(+)		(-)	(-)	(+)		(-)	
Other economic factors[2]				(+)				
CACFP:								
Unemployment rate	(-)	(-)	(-)	(-)	(+)	(+)	(+)	(+)
Program policy	(-)		(-)		(+/-)	(+)		

Source: USDA Economic Research Service calculations.

Notes: (+) = Expected effect is to increase participation. (-) = Expected effect is to decrease participation. (+)/(-) = Two changes occurred during the period with opposite expected effects of decreasing and increasing participation.

SNAP= Supplemental Nutrition Assistance Program; WIC = Special Supplemental Nutrition Program for Women, Infants, and Children; NSLP= National School Lunch Program; SBP= School Breakfast Program; CACFP= Child and Adult Care Food Program

[1] 2005 Gulf Coast Hurricanes.

[2] Low-skilled labor market conditions, such as real wages that underlie an increase in the poverty rate during a period of economic growth.

[3] Prior to the late 1990s, WIC was not fully funded and participation was rationed. Once WIC was fully funded, the unemployment rate started to impact participation.

APPENDIX A—SUPPLEMENTAL NUTRITION ASSISTANCE PROGRAM (SNAP) PARTICIPATION INFLUENCED BY ECONOMY AND POLICY: LITERATURE REVIEW

The literature on the relationship of SNAP participation with economic conditions and program policy dates back to work by Wertheimer and Fletcher (1985) and Dynaski et al. (1991), which used national quarterly data to estimate the impact of early program legislation (1977 through 1988) in conjunction with the effects of the unemployment rate and real wages on SNAP participation. In addition to finding that an increase in the unemploy- ment rate increases SNAP participation, both studies found that the Food Stamp Act of 1977 increased participation, while the Omnibus Budget Reconciliation Acts of 1981 reduced participation. Wertheimer and Fletcher (1985) also found that an increase in the poverty rate and a decrease in the real wage were associated with an increase in participation, while Dynaski (1991) found that the Hunger Prevention Act of 1988 increased participation.

The next round of studies used State variations in economic conditions and program policy, including welfare program policy, to estimate the dual impact of the economy and policy on SNAP participation during the 1993-2000 period of economic growth. This period was strongly influenced by welfare reform.[1] Kabbani and Wilde (2003) found that the fall in the unemployment rate explained 27 percent of the decline in participation, while State use of short certification periods and frequent recertification (e.g., every 3 months) explained 10 percent of the decline in participation. Kornfeld (2002) found that economic conditions explained 20 percent of the decline in participation, welfare reform (cross-program effects from changes to welfare programs) explained 21 percent, restricted eligibility for noncitizens and adults without dependents explained 10 percent, and SNAP reporting requirements (primarily short certification periods) explained 8 percent. Currie and Grogger (2001) found that unemployment explained 20 percent of the decline in caseloads, while welfare reform explained 30 percent. Klerman and Danielson (2011) found that economic conditions explained 31 percent of the change in participation and welfare reform explained 13 percent. They also found that the two SNAP policies of short certification—positive effect—and State replacement of paper coupons with Electronic Benefit Transfer (EBT)—negative effect—had offsetting effects on participation. In summarizing the findings of a few of the studies during this period, Hanson and Gunderson (2002) found that a 1-percentage-point increase in the unemployment rate would lead to a 700,000 to 1.5 million- person increase in SNAP participation after taking into account the influ- ence of program policy on SNAP participation.

Another set of studies, focusing on recent years, also used variation in State implementation of SNAP program policy options and variation in State unemployment rates to estimate the impact of the economy and policy on SNAP participation. During this time, SNAP offered States a number of policy options that would be expected to increase participation, in part as a response to low participation rates. Ratcliffe et al. (2008) found that the exclusion of a vehicle from the asset test for SNAP eligibility, longer certi- fication periods, expanded categorical eligibility, and State implementation of EBT all increased SNAP participation, while outreach spending had only a small lagged impact.[2] Mabli et al. (2009) found that a 1-percentage- point increase in the unemployment rate increased per capita participation (normalized by State population) by 3.7 percent, or 710,000 participants, after accounting for State population. SNAP policies that were found to increase participation were expanded categorical eligibility and simplified reporting for earners. Outreach spending was found to increase participation only when the unemployment rate was relatively low. Klerman and Danielson (2011) found that economic conditions explained 27 percent of the change in partici- pation, welfare policies explained 6 percent, and SNAP policies explained 16 percent. SNAP policies of significance for participants without cash welfare assistance were State implementation of EBT, vehicle exclusion, lengthening of certification periods, and expanded categorical eligibility (broad-based). SNAP participation for all persons except those who received SSI cash assis- tance increased by 5 percent after 1 year from a 1-percentage-point change in the unemployment rate, and an even greater increase occurred over a longer period for some household types.

Appendix B—Tables on Estimated Annual Average Change in Nutrition Assistance Program Participation

Appendix table 1. Estimated annual average change in Special Supplemental Nutrition Assistance Program (SNAP) participation

Appendix table 2. Estimated annual average change in Special Supplemental Nutrition Program for Women, Infants, and Children (WIC) participation

Appendix B, Table 1. Estimated annual average change in Special Supplemental Nutrition Assistance Program (SNAP) participation

Periods of economic growth (falling unemployment rate)	
1976 - 1979	
Thousand participants	147
Percent	1.2
1984 - 1989	
Thousand participants	-470
Percent	-2.3
1993 - 2000	
Thousand participants	-1,027
Percent	-4.6
1993 - 1994	
Thousand participants	1,034
Percent	4.0
1995 - 1996	
Thousand participants	-966
Percent	-3.6

Periods of economic growth (falling unemployment rate)	
1997 - 2000	
Thousand participants	-2,087
Percent	-9.4
2004 - 2007	
Thousand participants	1,267
Percent	5.6
Periods of economic decline (rising unemployment rate)	
1980 - 1983	
Thousand participants	993
Percent	5.6
1980 - 1981	
Thousand participants	2,389
Percent	12.9
1982 - 1983	
Thousand participants	-403
Percent	-1.8
1990 - 1992	
Thousand participants	2,200
Percent	10.6
2001 - 2003	
Thousand participants	1,352
Percent	7.4
2008 - 2010	
Thousand participants	4,662
Percent	15.4

Years shown are fiscal years.

Source: USDA Economic Research Service calculations based on USDA Food and Nutrition Service data.

Appendix B, Table 2. Estimated annual average change in Special Supplemental Nutrition Program for Women, Infants, and Children (WIC) participation

	Total participants	Women and infants	Children	Births
Periods of economic growth (falling unemployment rate)				
1976 - 1979				
Thousand participants	285	136	149	88
Percent	44.8	45.7	44.1	2.7
1984 - 1989				

Appendix B, Table 2. (Continued)

	Total participants	Women and infants	Children	Births
Thousand participants	264	157	107	67
Percent	8.6	9.8	7.4	1.8
1993 - 2000				
Thousand participants	224	91	132	-1
Percent	3.7	2.9	4.7	0.0
1993 - 1997				
Thousand participants	401	133	268	-37
Percent	6.5	4.2	9.1	-0.9
1998 - 2000				
Thousand participants	-72	23	-94	59
Percent	-1.0	0.6	-2.5	1.5
2004 - 2007				
Thousand participants	164	113	50	57
Percent	2.1	2.9	1.3	1.4
Periods of economic decline (rising unemployment rate)				
1980 - 1983				
Thousand participants	264	143	121	36
Percent	14.7	16.4	13.2	1.0
1990 - 1992				
Thousand participants	428	233	196	8
Percent	9.5	9.6	9.4	0.2
2001 - 2003				
Thousand participants	146	55	92	10
Percent	2.0	1.5	2.5	0.3
2008 - 2010				
Thousand participants	296	18	279	-103
Percent	3.5	0.4	6.5	-2.4
2008 - 2009				
Thousand participants	418	74	344	-93
Percent	4.9	1.7	8.2	-2.2
2010				
Thousand participants	53	-94	147	-124
Percent	0.6	-2.1	3.1	-3.0

Years shown are fiscal years.

Source: USDA Economic Research Service calculations based on USDA Food and Nutrition Service data.

Appendix B, Table 3. Estimated annual average change in National School Lunch Program (NSLP) participation

	Total participants	Free and reduced-price participants	Full price participants	Free and reduced-price as percent of total
Periods of economic growth (falling unemployment rate)				
1976 - 1979				
Thousand students	525	425	100	
Percent	2.0	4.1	0.7	2.0
1984 - 1989				
Thousand students	196	-87	283	
Percent	0.8	-0.7	2.4	-1.6
1993 - 2000				
Thousand students	337	317	21	
Percent	1.3	2.3	0.2	1.0
2004 - 2007				
Thousand students	530	371	159	
Percent	1.8	2.2	1.3	0.4
Periods of economic decline (rising unemployment rate)				
1980 - 1983				
Thousand students	-1,000	25	-1,025	
Percent	-3.8	0.4	-7.4	4.3
1990 - 1992				
Thousand students	144	542	-398	
Percent	0.6	4.6	-3.2	4.0
2001 - 2003				
Thousand students	362	341	21	
Percent	1.3	2.2	0.2	0.8
2008 - 2010				
Thousand students	357	845	-488	
Percent	1.2	4.5	-4.0	3.3

Years shown are fiscal years.

Source: USDA Economic Research Service calculations based on USDA Food and Nutrition Service data.

Appendix B, Table 4. Estimated annual average change in School Breakfast Program (SBP) participation

	Total participants	Free and reduced-price participants	Full price participants	Free and reduced-price as percent of total
Periods of economic growth (falling unemployment rate)				
1976 - 1979				
Thousand students	373	320	53	
Percent	16.2	16.8	13.7	0.6
1984 - 1989				
Thousand students	75	47	29	
Percent	2.1	1.5	7.1	-0.6
1993 - 2000				
Thousand students	329	253	76	
Percent	5.5	5.0	9.1	-0.5
2004 - 2007				
Thousand students	423	292	131	
Percent	4.7	4.0	7.9	-0.7
Periods of economic decline (rising unemployment rate)				
1980 - 1983				
Thousand students	13	63	-50	
Percent	0.7	2.5	-10.0	1.8
1990 - 1992				
Thousand students	369	337	31	
Percent	8.9	9.3	5.8	0.4
2001 - 2003				
Thousand students	292	207	85	
Percent	3.7	3.2	6.6	-0.5
2008 - 2010				
Thousand students	507	525	-19	
Percent	4.8	6.1	-0.9	1.3

Years shown are fiscal years.

Source: USDA Economic Research Service calculations based on USDA Food and Nutrition Service data.

Appendix B, Table 5. Estimated annual average change in Child and Adult Care Food Program (CACFP) participation

	Total participants	Free and reduced-price participants	Full price participants	Free and reduced-price as percent of total
Periods of economic growth (falling unemployment rate)				
1976 - 1979				
Thousand participants	56	37	19	
Percent	12.5	10.1	28.8	-2.2
1984 - 1989				
Thousand participants	75	61	14	
Percent	6.9	6.7	7.9	-0.2
1993 - 2000				
Thousand participants	113	90	22	
Percent	5.3	5.0	6.7	-0.3
2004 - 2007				
Thousand participants	73	43		
Percent	2.4	1.8	5.4	-0.6
Periods of economic decline (rising unemployment rate)				
1980 - 1983				
Thousand participants	81	75	6	
Percent	11.4	13.4	11.8	1.6
1990 - 1992				
Thousand participants	144	131	13	
Percent	9.6	10.4	5.5	0.7
2001 - 2003				
Thousand participants	70.0	52.3	17.7	
Percent	2.5	2.3	3.8	-0.3
2008 - 2010				
Thousand participants	48.7	48.3	0.4	
Percent	1.5	1.8	0.1	0.3

Years shown are fiscal years.

Source: USDA Economic Research Service calculations based on USDA Food and Nutrition Service data.

Appendix B, Table 6. Estimated annual average change in Supplemental Nutrition Assistance Program (SNAP) participation per 1-percentage-point change in unemployment rate

Periods of economic growth (falling unemployment rate)	
1976 - 1979	
Thousand participants	-266
Percent	-2.2
1984 - 1989	
Thousand participants	579
Percent	2.8
1993 - 2000	
Thousand participants	2,418
Percent	10.8
1993 - 1994	
Thousand participants	-1,900
Percent	-7.4
1995 - 1996	
Thousand participants	2,212
Percent	8.2
1997 - 2000	
Thousand participants	5,814
Percent	26.1
2004 - 2007	
Thousand participants	-3,468
Percent	-15.3
Periods of economic decline (rising unemployment rate)	
1980 - 1983	
Thousand participants	925
Percent	5.2
1980 - 1981	
Thousand participants	3,036
Percent	16.4
1982 - 1983	
Thousand participants	-296
Percent	-1.3
1990 - 1992	
Thousand participants	3,051
Percent	14.7
2001 - 2003	
Thousand participants	2,063

Periods of economic decline (rising unemployment rate)	
Percent	11.3
2008 - 2010	
Thousand participants	2,680
Percent	8.9

Years shown are fiscal years.

Source: USDA Economic Research Service calculations based on data from USDA Food and Nutrition Service and U.S. Department of Labor, Bureau of Labor Statistics.

Appendix B, Table 7. Estimated annual average change in Special Supplemental Nutrition Program for Women, Infants, and Children (WIC) participation per 1-percentage-point change in unemployment rate

	Total participants	Women and infants	Children
Periods of economic growth (falling unemployment rate)			
1998 - 2000			
Thousand participants	201	-64	265
Percent	2.7	-1.8	7.1
2004 - 2007			
Thousand participants	-448	-310	-137
Percent	-5.7	-7.8	-3.6
Periods of economic decline (rising unemployment rate)			
2001 - 2003			
Thousand participants	223	83	140
Percent	3.0	2.3	3.8
2008 - 2010			
Thousand participants	170	10	160
Percent	2.0	0.3	3.7
2008 - 2009			
Thousand participants	211	37	174
Percent	2.5	0.9	4.1
2010			
Thousand participants	42	-75	117
Percent	0.5	-1.7	2.5

Years shown are fiscal years.

Source: USDA Economic Research Service calculations based on data from USDA Food and Nutrition Service and U.S. Department of Labor, Bureau of Labor Statistics.

Appendix B, Table 8. Estimated annual average change in National School Lunch Program (NSLP) participation per 1-percentage-point change in unemployment rate

	Total participants	Free and reduced-price participants	Full price participants	Free and reduced-price as percent of total
Periods of economic growth (falling unemployment rate)				
1976 - 1979				
Thousand students	-948	-767	-181	
Percent	-3.7	-7.4	-1.2	-3.6
1984 - 1989				
Thousand students	-241	107	-349	
Percent	-1.0	0.9	-2.9	1.9
1993 - 2000				
Thousand students	-794	-746	-49	
Percent	-3.1	-5.4	-0.4	-0.4
2004 - 2007				
Thousand students	-1,452	-1,017	-435	
Percent	-5.0	-6.0	-3.6	-1.0
Periods of economic decline (rising unemployment rate)				
1980 - 1983				
Thousand students	-931	23	-954	
Percent	-3.6	0.3	-6.9	4.0
1990 - 1992				
Thousand students	200	752	-552	
Percent	0.8	6.4	-4.4	5.5
2001 - 2003				
Thousand students	553	521	32	
Percent	2.0	3.3	0.3	1.3
2008 - 2010				
Thousand students	205	486	-280	
Percent	0.7	2.6	-2.3	1.9

Years shown are fiscal years.

Source: USDA Economic Research Service calculations based on data from USDA Food and Nutrition Service and U.S. Department of Labor, Bureau of Labor Statistics.

Appendix B, Table 9. Estimated annual average change in School Breakfast Program (SBP) participation per 1-percentage point change in unemployment rate

	Total participants	Free and reduced-price participants	Full price participants	Free and reduced-price as percent of total
Periods of economic growth (falling unemployment rate)				
1976 - 1979				
Thousand students	-673	-578	-95	-1.0
Percent	-29.2	-30.4	-24.7	
1984 - 1989				
Thousand students	-93	-58	-35	
Percent	-2.6	-1.8	-8.8	0.8
1993 - 2000				
Thousand students	-776	-597	-179	
Percent	-13.0	-11.7	-21.4	1.3
2004 - 2007				
Thousand students	-1,159	-800	-359	
Percent	-12.8	-10.8	-21.7	1.9
Periods of economic decline (rising unemployment rate)				
1980 - 1983				
Thousand students	12	58	-47	1.7
Percent	0.7	2.3	-9.4	
1990 - 1992				
Thousand students	511	468	43	
Percent	12.3	13.0	8.0	0.6
2001 - 2003				
Thousand students	446	316	130	-0.8
Percent	5.7	4.8	10.0	
2008 - 2010				
Thousand students	291	302	-11	
Percent	2.7	3.5	-0.5	0.7

Years shown are fiscal years.

Source: USDA Economic Research Service calculations based on data from USDA Food and Nutrition Service and U.S. Department of Labor, Bureau of Labor Statistics.

Appendix B, Table 10. Estimated annual average change in Child and Adult Care Food Program (CACFP) participation per 1-percentage-point change in unemployment rate

	Total participants	Free and reduced-price participants	Full price participants	Free and reduced-price as percent of total
Periods of economic growth (falling unemployment rate)				
1976 - 1979				
Thousand participants	-101	-67	-34	
Percent	-22.6	-18.3	-52.1	4.0
1984 - 1989				
Thousand participants	-93	-76	-17	
Percent	-8.5	-8.3	-9.7	0.2
1993 - 2000				
Thousand participants	-266	-213	-53	
Percent	-12.4	-11.7	-15.8	0.6
2004 - 2007				
Thousand participants	-199	-119	-79	
Percent	-6.6	-4.8	-14.8	1.7
Periods of economic decline (rising unemployment rate)				
1980 - 1983				
Thousand participants	75	70	5	
Percent	10.6	12.5	11.0	1.5
1990 - 1992				
Thousand participants	200	182	18	
Percent	13.3	14.4	7.6	1.0
2001 - 2003				
Thousand participants	106.8	79.8	27.0	
Percent	3.9	3.5	5.9	-0.4
2008 - 2010				
Thousand participants	28.0	27.8	0.2	
Percent	0.9	1.1	0.0	0.2

Years shown are fiscal years.

Source: USDA Economic Research Service calculations based on data from USDA Food and Nutrition Service and U.S. Department of Labor, Bureau of Labor Statistics.

Appendix C—Child and Adult Care Food Program (CACFP) Total Participation

There have been three distinct phases of caseload growth in CACFP, distin- guished by changes in program legislation. The first phase, from 1976 to 1988, represents the expansion of a new program, with total participation increasing an average 9.8 percent (68,000 participants) per year. Prior to 1976, participation in the then-pilot program was targeted exclusively to center-based child care in poor areas (Hamilton et al., 2002). In 1975 legislation (P.L. 94-105), child care homes were allowed to participate in the program, and a three-level reimbursement structure was enacted based on the family income of the children receiving care, modeled after the National School Lunch Program. The Child Nutrition Amendments of 1978 (P.L. 95-627) permanently authorized the program. With the goal of increasing participation, the amendments also replaced the three-level reim- bursement structure in child care homes with a single reimbursement rate for all participants at a rate slightly below the free-meal reimbursement rate in child care centers. As a result of eliminating the means test for day care homes, more homes serving higher income children (those from families with incomes above 185 percent of the poverty guideline) participated in the program. Increased demand for child care also may have contributed to the program's growth during this period, as the labor force participa-tion rate of mothers with children under 6 years of age increased from 40.1 percent in 1976 to 56.1 percent in 1988 (U.S. Department of Labor, 2008).

A second phase of more rapid growth (in terms of the number of participants) from 1989 to 1996 may have been influenced by three successive legislative changes to the program (U.S. Department of Agriculture, 2011c). First, the Older Americans Act of 1987 (P.L. 100-175) authorized the participation of eligible adult day care centers; second, the Hunger Prevention Act of 1988 (P.L. 100-435) permitted an additional meal or snack for children in child care centers at least 8 hours per day; and, most important, the Child Nutrition and WIC Reauthorization Act of 1989 (P.L. 101-147) provided funds to expand family day care homes into low-income or rural areas, among other changes. During this period, there was once again a substantial increase in labor force participation by women with children under age 6: from 56.7 percent in 1989 to 62.3 percent in 1996 (U.S. Department of Labor, 2008). As a result, total participation increased an average 8.5 percent (143,500 partici-pants) per year during this phase.

Caseload growth in the third phase from 1997 to 2010 slowed down (in terms of the number of participants), back to that of the first phase. It began to slow after enactment of the Personal Responsibility and Work Opportunities Reconciliation Act of 1996 (PRWORA), which refocused the family child care component of the CACFP on low-income children by implementing a two-tiered reimbursement structure and lowering the maximum number of daily meals and snacks reimbursable in child care centers from four to three (U.S. Department of Agriculture, 2011c). Homes located in low-income areas or operated by persons with incomes at or below 185 percent of the Federal poverty guidelines were designated as Tier 1, and the meal reimburse-ment rates for Tier 1 homes were comparable to the rates that existed for all CACFP homes before the PRWORA. Tier 2 homes—family child care homes that did not meet the low-income criteria—received lower reimbursements, although the providers could be reimbursed at Tier 1 rates for children in their care whose family incomes were at or below 185 percent of the poverty guideline. The new rate structure took effect July 1, 1997, and the number of day care homes has decreased steadily since that time. However, the number of children in day care centers continued to increase, and overall participa- tion in the CACFP grew by an average 2.5 percent (72,000 participants) per year from 1997 to 2010. The annual average change in the number of partici- pants was similar to that in the first growth phase and half the number of the second growth phase.[1]

References

Bartlett, Susan, Melanie Brown-Lyons, Douglas Moore, and Angela Estacion.2000. "WIC Participant and Program Characteristics 1998." U.S. Department of Agriculture, Food and Nutrition Service, May.

Berry, Jeffrey M. 1984. *Feeding Hungry People: Rulemaking in the Food Stamp Program*. New Brunswick, NJ: Rutgers University Press.

Bitler, Marianne, Janet Currie, and John Karl Scholz. 2003. "WIC Eligibility and Participation," *Journal of Human Resources* 38 (supplement):1139-79.

Bivens, Josh, and John Irons. 2008. "A Feeble Recovery: The Fundamental Economic Weaknesses of the 2001-07 Expansion," Economic Policy Institute, Briefing Paper #214.

Blank, Rebecca. 2009. "Economic Change and the Structure of Opportunity for Less-Skilled Workers," in *Changing Poverty, Changing Policies*, Maria Cancian and Sheldon Danziger, eds. New York: Russell Sage Foundation.

Connor, Patty, Susan Bartlett, Michele Mendelson, Katherine Condon, and James Sutcliffe. 2010. "WIC Participant and Program Characteristics 2008." U.S. Department of Agriculture, Food and Nutrition Service, January.

Currie, Janet, and Jeffrey Grogger. 2001. "Explaining Recent Declines in Food Stamp Program Participation," in *Brookings-Wharton Papers on Urban Affairs*, W. G. Gale and J.R. Pack, eds. Washington, DC: Brookings Institution Press, pp. 203-29.

Devaney, Barbara, Linda Bilheimer, and Jennifer Schore. 1990. *The Savings in Medicaid Costs for Newborns and Their Mothers from Prenatal WIC Participation in the WIC Program: Volume 1,* U.S. Department of Agriculture, Food and Nutrition Service, October.

Dynaski, Mark, Anuradha Rangarajan, and Paul Decker. 1991. *Forecasting Food Stamp Program Participation and Benefits.* Prepared by Mathematica Policy Research, Inc. for U.S. Department of Agriculture, Food and Nutrition Service, August.

Greenstone, Michael, and Adam Looney. 2011. "What Is Happening to America's Less-Skilled Workers? The Importance of Education and Training in Today's Economy," Brookings Institution, Hamilton Project, Up-Front blog, December 2.

Hamilton, Brady E., Joyce A. Martin, and Stephanie J. Ventura. 2010. "Births: Preliminary data for 2009." *National Vital Statistics Report*, 59(3), December. National Center for Health Statistics. http://www.cdc.gov/nchs/data/nvsr/nvsr59/nvsr59_03.pdf.

Hamilton, William, Nancy Burstein, and Mary Kay Crepinsek. 2002. *Reimbursement Tiering in the CACFP: Summary Report to Congress on the Family Child Care Homes Legislative Changes Study.* Prepared by Abt Associates for the U.S. Department of Agriculture, Economic Research Service, Food Assistance and Nutrition Research Report No. 22, March.

Hanson, Kenneth, and Craig Gundersen. 2002. *Issues in Food Assistance: How Unemployment Affects the Food Stamp Program.* U.S. Department of Agriculture, Economic Research Service, FANRR 26-7, September.

Hanson, Kenneth, and Victor Oliveira. 2007. *The 2005 Gulf Coast Hurricanes' Effect on Food Stamp Program Caseloads and Benefits Issued.* U.S. Department of Agriculture, Economic Research Service, ERR-37, January.

Hoynes, Hilary. 2000. "The Employment, Earnings, and Income of Less-Skilled Workers over the Business Cycle," in *Finding Jobs: Work and Welfare Reform,* eds., David Card and Rebecca Blank. New York: Russell Sage Foundation.

Jackson, Kenneth, Phil Gleason, John Hall, and Rhonda Strauss. 2000. *Study of Direct Certification in the National School Lunch Program*. USDA, Food and Nutrition Service, CN-00-DC, September.

Kabbani, Nader, and Parke Wilde. 2003. "Short Recertification Periods in the U.S. Food Stamp Program," *Journal of Human Resources* 38(supplement):1112-38.

Klerman, Jacob Alex, and Caroline Danielson. 2011. "Transformation of the Supplemental Nutrition Assistance Program," *Journal of Policy Analysis and Management* 30(4):863-88.

Kornfeld, Robert. 2002. *Explaining Recent Trends in Food Stamp Program Caseloads*. Report prepared by Abt Associates, Inc. for the U.S. Department of Agriculture, Economic Research Service, E-FAN-02-008, March.

Mabli, James, Emily Sama Martin, and Laura Castner. 2009. *Effects of Economic Conditions and Program Policy on State Food Stamp Program Caseloads, 2000 to 2006*. U.S. Department of Agriculture, Economic Research Service, CCR-56, August.

McConnell, Sheena. 1991. *The Increase in Food Stamp Program Participation between 1989 and 1990: A Report to Congress*. Prepared by Mathematica Policy Research for the U.S. Department of Agriculture, Food and Nutrition Service, and submitted to the Committee on Appropriations, U.S. Senate, August.

McKernan, Signe-Mary, and Caroline Ratcliffe. 2003. *Employment Factors Influencing Food Stamp Program Participation*. U.S. Department of Agriculture, Economic Research Service, E-FAN-03-012, November.

Neftci, Salih. 1984. "Are Economic Time Series Asymmetric over the Business Cycle?" *Journal of Political Economy* 92(2), April:307-28.

Nord, Mark, and Mark Prell. 2011. *Food Security Improved Following the 2009 ARRA Increase in SNAP Benefits*. U.S. Department of Agriculture, Economic Research Service, ERR-116, April.

Ohls, James C., and Harold Beebout. 1993. *The Food Stamp Program: Design Tradeoffs, Policy, and Impacts*. Washington, DC: The Urban Institute Press.

Oliveira, Victor. 2011. *The Food Assistance Landscape, FY 2010 Annual Report*. U.S. Department of Agriculture, Economic Research Service, EIB 6-8, March.

Ratcliffe, Caroline, Signe-Mary McKerman, and Kenneth Finegold. 2008. "Effects of Food Stamp and TANF Policies on Food Stamp Receipt," *Social Service Review* 82:291-334.

Sichel, Daniel. 1993. "Business Cycle Asymmetry: A Deeper Look," *Economic Inquiry* 31(2), April:224-36.

Schreft, Stacey, Arati Singh, and Ashley Hodgson. 2005. "Jobless Recoveries and the Wait-and-See Hypothesis," Federal Reserve Bank of Kansas City, Economic Review, 4th Quarter.

Sutton, Paul, and Brady Hamilton. 2011. "Recent Trends in Births and Fertility Rates through 2010." NCHS Health E-Stat, National Center for Health Statistics, June.

Swann, Christopher A. 2010. "WIC Eligibility and Participation: The Roles of Changing Policies, Economic Conditions, and Demographics," *The B. E. Journal of Economic Analysis & Policy*, 10(1), Article 21.

Trippe, Carole, Liz Schott, Nancy Wemmerus, and Andrew Burwick. 2004. *Simplified Reporting and Transitional Benefits in the Food Stamp Program: Case Studies of State Implementation.* Prepared by Mathematica Policy Research for U.S. Department of Agriculture, Economic Research Service, E-FAN-04-003, May.

U.S. Department of Agriculture, Food and Nutrition Service. 2001. *The Decline in Food Stamp Participation: A Report to Congress*, July.

U.S. Department of Agriculture, Food and Nutrition Service. 2010a. *Characteristics of Supplemental Nutrition Assistance Program Households: Fiscal Year 2009*, October.

U.S. Department of Agriculture, Food and Nutrition Service. 2010b. *Direct Certification in the National School Lunch Program: State Implementation Progress School Year 2009–2010.* Report CN-10-DC, October.

U.S. Department of Agriculture, Food and Nutrition Service. 2010c. *Supplemental Nutrition Assistance Program State Options Report, Ninth Edition,* November.

U.S. Department of Agriculture, Food and Nutrition Service. 2011a. "SNAP: Program Policy, Legislation." Accessed April 2011. http://www.fns.usda.gov/snap/rules/Legislation/default.htm.

U.S. Department of Agriculture, Food and Nutrition Service. 2011b. *Trends in Supplemental Nutrition Assistance Program Participation Rates: Fiscal Year 2002 to Fiscal Year 2009*, August.

U.S. Department of Agriculture, Food and Nutrition Service. 2011c. "CACFP: Legislative History." Accessed April 2011. http://www.fns.usda.gov/cnd/care/history.htm.

U.S. Department of Agriculture, Office of Communications. 1996. *Agricultural Fact Book 1996.* See chapter 8, Food, Nutrition, and Consumer Services; section on School Breakfast Program.

U.S. Department of Labor, U.S. Bureau of Labor Statistics. 2008. *Women in the Labor Force: A Databook (2008 edition)*, Report 1011, December.

U.S. General Accounting Office. 1984. *Participation in the National School Lunch Program: Report to the Chairman, Committee on Agriculture, Nutrition, and Forestry, United States Senate*, GAO/RCED-84-132, March 30.

U.S. General Accounting Office. 1992. *Early Intervention: Federal Investments Like WIC Can Produce Savings*, GAO/HRD-92-18, April.

U.S. Government Accountability Office. 1999. *Food Stamp Program: Various Factors Have Led to Declining Participation*, GAO/RCED-99-185, July.

U.S. Government Accountability Office. 2002. *Food Stamp Program: State's Use of Options and Waivers to Improve Program Administration and Promote Access*, GAO-02-409, February.

U.S. Government Accountability Office. 2004. *Food Stamp Program: Steps Have Been Taken to Increase Participation of Working Families*, GAO-04-346, March.

U.S. Government Accountability Office. 2009. *School Meal Programs: Experiences of the States and Districts that Eliminated Reduced-Price Fees*, GAO-09-584, July.

Wertheimer, Richard, and Thaddeus Fletcher. 1985. *Analysis of Interactions between the Macroeconomy and Food Stamp Program Changes.* Prepared by Urban Institute and Data Resources, Inc. for U.S. Department of Agriculture, Food and Nutrition Service, October.

Zedlewski, Sheila, and Amelia Gruber. 2001. *Former Welfare Families Continue to Leave the Food Stamp Program*, Assessing the New Federalism Discussion Paper 01-05. Washington, DC: The Urban Institute, March.

Zedlewski, Sheila, and Kelly Rader. 2004. *Recent Trends in Food Stamp Participation among Poor Families with Children*, Assessing the New Federalism Discussion Paper 04-03. Washington, DC: The Urban Institute, June.

Zedlewski, Sheila, David Wittenburg, Carolyn O'Brien, Robin Koralek, Sandra Nelson, and Gretchen Rowe. 2005. *Evaluation of Food Stamp Research Grants to Improve Access Through New Technology and Partnerships.* Prepared by The Urban Institute for U.S. Department of Agriculture, Food and Nutrition Service, September.

End Notes

[1] As discussed in the data and meth- odology section, dates for the growth and decline phases of the business cycles in this report differ somewhat from the dates for the turning points in the business cycles specified by the National Bureau of Economic Research (NBER).

[2] The use of annual, national-level data on program participation provides a common framework for the analysis of programs with different lengths of operation (e.g., the school programs operate on a 9-month school year). The use of monthly, State-level data would allow for a more precise quantitative estimation of the relationship between economic conditions and program participation for some programs. For our exploratory analysis, however, the averaging of State monthly data on participation and unemployment into annual national measures allows for multiyear trends over the busi- ness cycle to be more transparent and illustrative of the basic relationship between program participation and economic conditions.

[3] Throughout the report, the terms "participation" and "caseloads" are used interchangeably in reference to the annual average number of program participants (persons).

[4] The Business Cycle Dating Committee of the NBER determines the dates of recessions, which they define as a significant decline in economic activity lasting more than a few months and normally visible in real Gross Domestic Product (GDP), real income, employment, industrial production, and real sales. The NBER dates of recessions are: November 1973 to March 1975; January 1980 to November 1982 (which includes the two recession periods of January to July 1980 and July 1981 to November 1982); July 1990 to March 1991; March 2001 to November 2001; and December 2007 to June 2009.

[5] Population growth does not appear to have had a significant influence on SNAP participation at the national level, so this study does not include population as a factor in the analysis. Over the study period, average popula- tion growth was relatively stable, 1 percent per year, with a minimum of 0.7 percent and a maximum of 1.3 percent per year. If population growth had a significant effect on SNAP participation, there should be an upward trend around which the cyclical pattern caused by economic conditions occurred. Such an upward trend does not appear to be signifi- cant. Participation has been cyclical around a fairly flat midpoint of 20 to 25 million persons. The 1994 peak in caseloads was not exceeded until 2008, while the 2001 low was the lowest since 1977. The rise in participation during the 2000s was related more to economic conditions and program policy than population growth.

[6] Recipients paid an amount commensurate with the normal food expenditures for their household size and income and received that amount plus an additional amount of food stamps to "more nearly obtain" a low-cost, nutritionally adequate diet for that household size (Food Stamp Act of 1964, P.L 88-525; Berry, 1984). The bonus amount ranged from 100 percent to 20 percent of the total value of food stamps, depending on house- hold income. In setting the purchase price and bonus amount, there was an attempt to balance concern for trafficking excess benefits and for providing an incentive to purchase an adequate diet.

[7] Among other changes, the 1981 and 1982 legislation set a gross income eligibility standard at 130 percent of poverty for households without elderly or disabled members in addition to the net income test at 100 percent of poverty, lowered the earned income deduction from 20 to 18 percent, and required States to implement peri- odic reporting (U.S. Department of Agriculture, 2011a).

[8] The 1985 legislation made house- holds in which all members receive Aid to Families with Dependent Children (AFDC) or Supplemental Security Income (SSI) categorically eligible

for SNAP; raised the earned income deduction from 18 to 20 percent; raised the shelter deduction limit and dependent-care deduction; raised the asset limit from $1,500 to $2,000; and authorized simplified application for households in which at least one member receives AFDC, SSI, or Medicaid. Policy changes in the 1988 legislation include raising the maximum benefit amount above 100 percent of the Thrifty Food Plan cost; providing greater State flex- ibility in design of the application form to make it easier to use; requiring States to be clearer about necessary reporting responsibility and docu- mentation; requiring States to provide prompt and accurate certification; and improving the method for claiming recurring medical expenses for the medical deduction (U.S. Department of Agriculture, 2011a).

[9] Chapter 3 of the 1993 Act (Mickey Leland Childhood Hunger Relief Act) made various changes to program policy that would have eased eligibility rules and increased the take-up rate, including an incremental increase to the shelter deduction cap; excluding earned income tax credit as resources for 12 months from receipt; disre- garding child support payments as income to the payer; increasing the degree to which vehicles are disre- garded as assets; revising the defi- nition of a food stamp household; and increasing the degree to which dependent care expense deductions can be claimed (U.S. Department of Agriculture, 2011a).

[10] The empirical studies for this period discussed in appendix A did not include this national policy change in the analysis of SNAP participation.

[11] Welfare reform eliminated eligibility of most legal immigrants, placed time limits on SNAP receipt for able-bodied adults without dependents (ABAWDs) who are not working, and reduced maximum benefit amount to 100 percent of the Thrifty Food Plan cost. Subsequent budget legislation in 1997 and 1998 restored eligibility to some legal immigrants and allowed States to exempt up to 15 percent of ABAWDs (U.S. Department of Agriculture, 2011a).

[12] Welfare reform replaced the Nation's welfare program for low- income families (Aid to Families with Dependent Children, AFDC) with the Temporary Assistance for Needy Families (TANF) program. Among other changes, the act required States to have a minimum percentage of welfare households working or participating in work-related activities. To meet these requirements, welfare recipients and new applicants were provided incentives to move into the workforce and off the welfare program; consequently caseloads fell dramati- cally. Even if the households leaving welfare remained eligible for SNAP, many did not remain on or apply for SNAP benefits.

[13] The Agriculture Appropriations Act of 2001 (P.L. 106-387) expanded outreach and allowed use of TANF vehicle limits. The options of simpli- fied reporting, transitional benefits, and expanded categorical eligibility were allowed through USDA-FNS regula- tions. Households are categorically eligible for SNAP when they partici- pate (receive cash or noncash benefits) in TANF or receive General Assistance (GA) or Supplemental Security Income (SSI), without having to meet the SNAP asset limits or the gross and net income eligibility standards. However, SNAP benefits are still calculated on the basis of household income (U.S. Department of Agriculture, 2010a).

[14] The empirical studies on SNAP participation for the 2004-07 period (appendix A) did not explicitly account for these labor market conditions in their analysis. They focused on unem- ployment rates (current and lagged), program policy, and State minimum wages. The lagged unemployment rates could have been a proxy for the poor labor market conditions that persisted even though the current unemployment rate was falling.

[15] The 2-to-3 million change in participation per 1-percentage-point change in the unemployment rate is larger than the estimated impacts found in some of the studies reviewed in appendix A. In part, the differ- ence can be attributed to the change in participation due to changes in program policy that were accounted for in the empirical studies and by the fact that the empirical studies only account for about half of the change in participation.

[16] For example, a study by Devaney et al. (1990), based on 1987-88 data from five States, found that each dollar spent on prenatal WIC services yielded a $1.77 to $3.13 savings in Medicaid costs for newborns and mothers over the first 60 days after birth. The U.S. General Accounting Office (1992) statisti-cally combined results from 17 studies conducted between 1971 and 1988 that compared rates of low birthweight among WIC participants and similar nonparticipants and concluded that "each Federal dollar invested in WIC benefits returns an estimated $3.50 over 18 years in discounted present value."

[17] There is some year-to-year varia- tion with the annual average increase in monthly participation. Of particular note is the relatively small increase in participation from 1981 to 1982 (fig. 6) due to the Omnibus Budget Reconciliation Act of 1981, which restrained the growth of funding to WIC and other programs to slow the growth of Government spending and reduce the budget deficit.

[18] Also in 1989, legislation was enacted that established adjunct eligibility to recipients of food stamps, Medicaid, and Aid to Families with Dependent Children (AFDC), with the intent of simplifying the WIC applica-tion process. Swann (2010) attributes the increase in WIC participation from 1983 to 2006 in part to expansions in Medicaid. However, the impact of Medicaid expansion may be overstated as the study did not take into account the effect that the implementation of infant formula rebates had on the increase in WIC participation. The study also did not consider that for much of the study period WIC was not fully funded and participation was rationed. When the legislation was implemented in 1989, the income eligibility criterion for Medicaid was lower than the 185 percent of poverty for WIC. Subsequently, some States now enable people with income above 185 percent of poverty to enroll in Medicaid and, therefore, to be eligible for WIC. However, administrative data for 1992 to 2008 show that during this period, at most only 2 percent of WIC partici-pants had income above 185 percent of poverty (Connor et al., (2010)).

[19] The number of women and infants participating in WIC track closely and are combined in our analysis.

[20] WIC regulations allow for considerable flexibility in how WIC agencies interpret the period used in determining an applicant's income eligibility. WIC State agencies may "consider the income of the family during the past 12 months and the family's current income to determine which indicator more accurately reflects the family's status" (7 CFR 246.7). Women are less likely to be working in the period shortly before and after a birth, and therefore are more likely to meet the program's income eligibility requirements based on the family's "current" income.

[21] During 2009, States implemented revisions to the food packages that provided WIC participants with a wider variety of food and WIC State agencies with greater flexibility in prescribing food packages for participants with cultural food preferences. These changes in the composition of the WIC food packages may have had an effect on participation in 2010, but it is unclear in what direction and to what degree.

[22] In this report, students receiving free lunches and students receiving reduced-price lunches were combined into one group. In recent years, some States and school districts have eliminated the reduced-price fee for break- fast and/or lunch and have provided free meals to children eligible for reduced-price meals. These programs are known as elimination of

reduced- price fee (ERP) programs. The U.S. Government Accountability Office (2009) identified at least 5 Statewide ERP programs (CO, ME, MN, VT, and WA) and 35 district-level programs in 19 other States during the school year 2008-09.

[23] Program participation refers to the average daily number of participants.

[24] The 1981 Act also raised the income limit for free lunches from 125 to 130 percent of poverty and lowered the limit for reduced-price lunches from 195 to 185 percent of poverty (U.S. General Accounting Office, 1984). In response to the change in income limits, some students moved into a price category requiring them to pay more for lunch while others paid less, with the net effect on the percent of students receiving free and reduced- price meals unclear.

[25] The Child Nutrition and WIC Reauthorization Act of 2004 contained another provision potentially affecting the determination of free and reduced- price meal eligibility. Prior to the provision, households with children receiving free or reduced-price meals were required to report changes in circumstances that could affect their eligibility, such as an increase in income of $50 per month ($600 annually), a decrease in household size, or when the household was no longer certified eligible for food stamps or Temporary Assistance for Needy Families (TANF). Beginning with school year 2004-05, children were certified for the school year and up to 30 days into the next school year. It is not known to what degree, if any, this provision affected the percentage of NSLP participants receiving free and reduced-price meals.

[26] The Act of 1981 reduced the Federal reimbursement rates paid to schools for both full-price and reduced- price breakfasts. As a result, the number of participants receiving full-price meals fell while the number receiving free and reduced-price meals rose, although by an amount smaller than would be expected during an economic decline (appendix B, table 4).

[27] Meals served at day care homes with Tier I and Tier II reimbursement are treated as free and reduced-price meals. The data for CACFP pertain to the percent of meals that are free and reduced-price, while the data for the other child nutrition programs (NSLP and SBP) pertain to the number and percent, of participants (children in schools) who receive free and reduced- price meals.

End Notes for Appendix A

[1] The Personal Responsibility and Work Opportunity Reconciliation Act of 1996 (welfare reform) replaced the Nation's welfare program for low- income families (Aid to Families with Dependent Children, AFDC) with the Temporary Assistance for Needy Families (TANF) program, which offered States more control over the design of their State welfare system. Some of the TANF options that States used had cross-program effects on participation in SNAP. In the empirical studies of SNAP participation, welfare reform policies refer to these cross- program effects. Welfare reform also made changes to SNAP that tightened eligibility rules and reduced benefits, such as restricted eligibility for noncitizens and adults without dependents who are not working. In the empirical studies, the SNAP policy changes were either treated as separate polices or not at all since they were largely national policy changes.

[2] Categorical eligibility eliminates the requirement for valuation of vehi- cles and other assets and the applica- tion of the resource test in determining eligibility. Most States have established categorical eligibility through "broad- based" eligibility requirements (such as making

brochures available in certi- fication offices or including informa- tion/800 numbers about other available programs on SNAP applications); other States have established categorical eligibility through "narrow" eligi-bility requirements (e.g., requiring the client to be actually enrolled in certain programs such as employment assistance or to be receiving child care or transportation assistance); and a few States have established categorical eligibility through the requirement that applicants receive cash assistance from a means-tested welfare program (U.S. Department of Agriculture, Food and Nutrition Service, 2010c).

End Notes for Appendix C

[1] During the third phase, the labor force participation rate of mothers with children under 6 decreased slightly, from 65 percent in 1997 to 63.5 percent in 2007 (U.S. Department of Labor, 2008).

In: Economic Conditions ...
Editor: Oscar Gutierrez

ISBN: 978-1-62417-520-6

Chapter 2

DOMESTIC FOOD ASSISTANCE: SUMMARY OF PROGRAMS*

Randy Alison Aussenberg and Kirsten J. Colello

SUMMARY

Over the years, Congress has authorized and the federal government has administered programs to provide food to the hungry and to other vulnerable populations in this country. This report offers a brief overview of hunger and food insecurity along with the related network of programs. The report is structured around three main tables that contain information about each program, including its authorizing language, administering agency, eligibility, services provided, participation data, and funding information. In between the tables, contextual information about this policy area and program administration is provided that may assist Congress in tracking developments in domestic food assistance. This report provides a bird's-eye view of domestic food assistance and can be used both to learn about the details of individual programs as well as compare and contrast features across programs.

This report includes overview information for the U.S. Department of Agriculture's Food and Nutrition Service (USDA-FNS) Programs as well as nutrition programs administered by the U.S. Department of Health and Human Services' Administration on Aging (HHS-AOA). USDA-FNS programs include nutrition programs authorized in the 2008 farm

* This is an edited, reformatted and augmented version of Congressional Research Service, Publication No. R42353, dated February 13, 2012.

bill (the Food, Conservation, and Energy Act of 2008; P.L. 110-246). Programs included in the farm bill are the Supplemental Nutrition Assistance Program (SNAP), Emergency Food Assistance Program (TEFAP), Commodity Supplemental Food Program (CSFP), Fresh Fruit and Vegetable Program, and the Senior Farmers' Market Nutrition Program. USDA-FNS also administers programs not contained in the farm bill: the Special Supplemental Nutrition Program for Women, Infants, and Children (WIC) and Child Nutrition programs (School Breakfast Program, National School Lunch Program (NSLP), Summer Food Service Program (SFSP), Special Milk Program, and Child and Adult Care Food Program (CACFP)). HHS-AOA programs are the nutrition programs contained in the Older Americans Act (OAA)—Congregate Nutrition Program; Home Delivered Nutrition Program; Grants to Native Americans: Supportive and Nutrition Services; and the Nutrition Service Incentive Program (NSIP).

BACKGROUND

This report gives an overview of the federal programs that provide food assistance within the United States and the territories. The report begins by discussing common concepts and themes across the network of domestic food assistance programs. The report is split into two main parts: programs administered by the U.S. Department of Agriculture's Food and Nutrition Service (USDA-FNS), and programs administered by the U.S. Department of Health and Human Services' Administration on Aging (HHS-AOA). Within the USDA-FNS section are two subsections of programs: Farm Bill programs (Table 1), and the Special Supplemental Nutrition Program for Women, Infants, and Children (WIC) and Child Nutrition Programs (Table 2). Within the HHS-AOA section, Table 3 provides an overview of the Older Americans Act nutrition programs.[1] The tables within this report are intended to provide summary information, which can help illustrate the ways in which domestic food assistance programs are both similar and different.

Hunger and Food Insecurity

Congress has long been interested in issues of hunger and allocating federal resources to address hunger in this country. The federal programs discussed in this report pursue the goal of providing food to low-income and needy populations, seeking to prevent hunger. Some of these programs, such as the National School Lunch Program, have deep roots dating to the Depression era.

Evaluating trends in hunger in our nation is crucial to understanding if the efforts to prevent hunger are working and in recognizing if there are particular vulnerable populations that need assistance. Hunger, however, is a challenging concept to measure. For that reason, the terms "food security" and "food insecurity," as opposed to "hunger," are the prevailing terms used to describe the ability to access adequate food.

"Food security" and "food insecurity" focus on those economic and other access-related reasons associated with an individual's ability to purchase or otherwise obtain enough to eat. They are also terms that can be objectively measured. For this reason, a 2006 panel convened by the National Research Council, at the request of USDA, reviewed USDA measurements related to food adequacy. The panel recommended that USDA make a clear distinction between food insecurity and hunger. According to the panel, hunger is an individual-level physiological condition that is not feasible to measure through a household survey.[2] Furthermore, the panel stated that it is difficult to capture gradations in hunger through individual assessment. Thus, the terms food security and food insecurity do not capture those non-economic or other individual behaviors that may result in the physical condition of being hungry. For example, these terms do not capture instances where an individual may have missed a meal due to illness or because they were otherwise too busy to eat.

Each year, the U.S. Department of Agriculture's Economic Research Service (USDA-ERS) conducts an analysis based on Current Population Survey (CPS) data to measure food security in the United States.[3] ERS uses terminology that indicates whether a household was able to purchase or otherwise acquire enough to eat in 2010 ("food security") or not able to purchase or acquire enough to eat ("food insecurity"). Since 2006, ERS has distinguished between a spectrum of four levels of food security, listed below from highest to lowest:

High food security—Households had no problems, or anxiety about, consistently accessing adequate food. [This is a subcategory of food *security*.]

Marginal food security—Households had problems at times, or anxiety about, accessing adequate food, but the quality, variety, and quantity of their food intake were not substantially reduced. [This is a subcategory of food *security*.]

Low food security—Households reduced the quality, variety, and desirability of their diets, but the quantity of food intake and normal eating patterns were not substantially disrupted. [This is a subcategory of food *insecurity*.]

Very low food security—At times during the year, eating patterns of one or more household members were disrupted and food intake reduced because the household lacked money and other resources for food. [This is a subcategory of food *insecurity*.][4]

Findings from the USDA-ERS report on 2010 food security[5] include the following rates of food security and food insecurity among U.S households:

- 14.5% of U.S. households were *food insecure* throughout 2010 (85.5% of U.S. households were *food secure*). This was not a statistically significant difference from 2009 rates, which were 14.6% and 85.4%, respectively.
- 5.4% had *very low food security*; about one-third of all food insecure households have very low food security. This is a statistically significant reduction from the 2009 rate of 5.7%. Declines (reduction in food insecurity) were greatest for households with children, women living alone, and households with annual income below 185% of the poverty line.
- 7.9% of households that included an elderly member were *food insecure*. This rate is not a statistically significant change from the 2009 rate of 9.5%.
- 59% of *food insecure* households reported that they had participated in the Supplemental Nutrition Assistance (SNAP), WIC, or National School Lunch Program in the last month.

Program Variation

There are a number of domestic food assistance programs. Although each of the 17 programs discussed in this report provides for food in some way, the ways in which each program accomplishes this goal vary. For example, programs vary with respect to the target population (e.g., pregnant women, children, older individuals), eligibility requirements, and types of assistance provided (e.g., commodity foods versus prepared meals), In an April 2011 report, the Government Accountability Office (GAO) listed 70 programs that pertain to food and nutrition but ultimately narrowed their study to a smaller subset of programs that focus on food assistance or coordination of food assistance activities.[6]

One way to examine this variation is to compare the eligible populations for these domestic food assistance programs. For instance, the WIC program is available to children under the age of 5, while the school meals programs (National School Lunch Program, School Breakfast Program) become available to school-age children. Another way to examine this variation is to examine the benefits that programs provide. Within this constellation of programs, federal resources provide benefits redeemable for uncooked foods, cash assistance to support program operations, USDA-purchased commodity foods (discussed further in the next section), and prepared meals. While some programs provide specific foods (for example, through the federal and state requirements for "food package" in the Commodity Supplemental Food Program and WIC), the Supplemental Nutrition Assistance Program (SNAP) gives benefits that may be redeemed for a wide variety of foods at authorized retailers. OAA programs provide prepared meals that not only assist those who lack adequate resources to purchase food, but can also assist those who lack the functional capacity to prepare a meal on their own.

The following sections of the report and the accompanying tables provide more details about the services, eligibility, participation, and funding for each program. They help illustrate the similarities and differences between the programs, including the extent to which they provide similar or distinct forms of assistance to similar or distinct populations.

USDA-FNS PROGRAMS

USDA's Food and Nutrition Service (FNS) administers domestic food assistance programs authorized in the farm bill (**Table 1**),[7] as well as WIC and Child Nutrition Programs (**Table 2**). **Table 1** and **Table 2** provide details on the USDA-FNS programs, including services provided, eligibility, participation, and funding.

The USDA-FNS national office works in concert with USDA's regional offices[8] and state agencies. With respect to SNAP (formerly known as the Food Stamp Program), state agencies and legislatures have a number of options and waivers that can affect SNAP program operations from state to state. USDA-FNS's "SNAP State Options" report illustrates how states are administering the program. [9] With respect to school meals programs (National School Lunch Program and School Breakfast Program), state departments of education and school districts play a role in administering these programs. WIC as well as the Child and Adult Care Food Program (CACFP) are often co-administered by state and local health departments.

USDA Food Assistance Resources

- USDA-FNS Website: http://www.fns.usda.gov/ fns/—Program descriptions, press releases, current policy guidance and regulations, and participation and spending data. Information is organized into SNAP, WIC, School Meals, Food Distribution, and other child nutrition programs.
- USDA-FNS Office of Research and Analysis: http://www.fns.usda.gov/ora/—USDA sponsored data, research, and analysis on the participation and effectiveness of USDA-FNS programs.
- USDA's Economic Research Service (ERS) Food and Nutrition Assistance Products: http://www.ers.usda.gov/Browse/view.aspx?subject=FoodNutritionAssistance—ERS provides research on questions of food insecurity as well as program-specific questions.

As mentioned above, USDA commodity[10] foods are foods purchased by the USDA for distribution to USDA nutrition programs. The programs in this report that include USDA commodity foods are The Emergency Food Assistance Program (TEFAP), Commodity Supplemental Food Program (CSFP), National School Lunch Program (NSLP), Summer Food Service Program (SFSP), and Child and Adult Care Food Program (CACFP). USDA commodity foods are also provided to the HHS-AOA's Nutrition Services Incentive Program (NSIP) (**Table 3**). These programs distribute "entitlement commodities" (an amount of USDA foods to which grantees are entitled by law) as well as "bonus commodities" (USDA food purchases based on requests from the agricultural producer community).[11]

These domestic food assistance programs have a historical, and in most respects, ongoing relationship with farming and agriculture. For example, the first Food Stamp Program, a pilot program in the 1940's, sold orange and blue "food stamps" to program participants.[12] While $1 would provide a program participant with $1 in value of "orange stamps" that could be spent on any food, the program participant would also receive an additional 50 cents worth of "blue stamps," which could only be used to purchase agricultural products that were in surplus. Commodity donation programs that supported the post-

Depression farm economy were precursors to the National School Lunch Program.[13] TEFAP and several of the child nutrition programs still benefit from USDA commodity foods as well as USDA's donation of bonus commodities, which USDA purchases based on agricultural producers' identification of surplus goods or need for price support. As a contemporary example, the 2008 farm bill (P.L. 110-246), USDA initiatives, and current legislative proposals include efforts to promote "farm-to-school" endeavors, seeking, for example, to facilitate school cafeterias' purchasing from local and regional farms.[14]

Farm Bill

Table 1 lists those programs that were most recently reauthorized in the 2008 farm bill. The "farm bill" is an omnibus reauthorization and extension of dozens of farm, food, and nutrition laws. Most recently, Congress passed the Food, Conservation and Energy Act of 2008 (P.L. 110- 246), which is referred to as the 2008 farm bill. The 2008 farm bill included 15 titles on topics ranging from conservation, rural development, and research to horticulture.[15] The nutrition title, Title IV, included all of the programs listed in Table 1.

Farm bill nutrition programs have their authorizing language in the

- Food and Nutrition Act of 2008 (originally P.L. 95-113, most recently amended by P.L. 111-296),
- Emergency Food Assistance Act of 1983 (originally P.L. 98-8, most recently amended by P.L. 110-246), and
- Agriculture Consumer and Protection Act of 1973 (originally P.L. 93-86, most recently amended by P.L. 110-246).

The primary food assistance program in the farm bill is the Supplemental Nutrition Assistance Program (SNAP). The Congressional Budget Office (CBO) found that close to 75% of the 2008 farm bill spending was in the nutrition title, Title IV. This is primarily due to the mandatory money associated with SNAP. Formerly referred to as the Food Stamp Program, the federal program name change to SNAP was included in the 2008 farm bill.

Farm bill nutrition programs are under the jurisdiction of the House Agriculture Committee and the Senate Committee on Agriculture and Forestry.[16] The 2008 farm bill is set to expire at the end of FY2012.

WIC and Child Nutrition Programs

Table 2 lists the programs authorized by the Richard B. Russell National School Lunch Act (P.L. 79-396) and the Child Nutrition Act of 1966 (P.L. 108-269). Broadly, the programs contained in these laws are the Special Supplemental Nutrition Program for Women, Infants, and Children (WIC) as well as the "child nutrition programs." "Child nutrition programs" is a category used to describe the USDA-FNS programs that help to provide food for children in school or institutional settings. The National School Lunch and School Breakfast programs provide a per-meal subsidy for each meal that is served for free, for a reduced-price, or for a full-price (called a "paid" meal). The Child and Adult Care Food Program (CACFP) and Summer Food Service Program (SFSP) will, under certain circumstances, provide free meals or snacks to all the children at a site, because it is the site (not the child) that is subject to eligibility criteria. The Fresh Fruit and Vegetable Program (FFVP), or snack program (see Table 1), is sometimes referred to as a child nutrition program. In this report, it is included in farm bill programs because FFVP was included in the 2008 farm bill. Generally, the WIC and Child Nutrition Programs are reauthorized for a five-year period. The most recent reauthorization, the Healthy, Hunger-Free Kids Act of 2010 (P.L. 111-296), was signed into law in December 2010. It reauthorized these programs through FY2015. The 112th Congress may have an interest in oversight as USDA promulgates rules, releases guidance, and otherwise implements the legislation.

Resources for Tracking the Implementation of the Healthy, Hunger-Free Kids Act of 2010 (P.L. 111-296)

USDA Resources:

- USDA-FNS keeps a clearinghouse of Healthy, Hunger-Free Kids Act of 2010 resources and implementation updates on the web: http://www.fns.usda.gov/cnd/Governance/Legislation/CNR_2010.htm
- USDA-FNS's anticipated timeline for implementation can be found here: http://www.fns.usda.gov/cnd/Governance/Legislation/ implementation_actions.pdf.

Federal Register—https://www.federalregister.gov/topics/nutrition—The *Federal Register* allows you to browse by topic. The nutrition listing, while not exclusively child nutrition or P.L. 111-296 news, gives a glimpse of related notices.

Table 1. Overview of Farm Bill Programs

Authorizing Legislation / Federal Administrative Entity	Program Information	FY2012 Funding (in millions)[a]
Supplemental Nutrition Assistance Program (SNAP, formerly the Food Stamp Program)		
Food and Nutrition Act (7 U.S.C. 2011 et seq.) / Administered by the U.S. Department of Agriculture's Food and Nutrition Service (USDA-FNS)	**Description**: Provides benefits (through the use of electronic benefit transfer cards) that supplement lowincome recipients' food purchasing power. Benefits vary by household size, income, and expenses (like shelter and medical costs) and currently average $133 per person per month. In lieu of SNAP benefits, (1) Puerto Rico operates a nutrition assistance block grant program using rules very similar to SNAP; (2) over 250 Indian reservations operate a food distribution program (Food Distribution Program on Indian Reservations (FDPIR)) with eligibility rules close to SNAP; and (3) American Samoa and the Northern Marianas receive nutrition assistance block grants for programs serving their low-income populations. **Eligibility:** In general, eligible households must meet a gross income test (monthly cash income below 130% of the federal poverty guidelines), net income (monthly cash income subtracting SNAP deductible expenses at or below 100% of the federal poverty guidelines), liquid assets under $2,000 (assets under $3,000 if elderly or disabled household members). However, households with elderly or disabled members do not have to meet the gross income test. Recipients of Temporary Assistance for Needy Families (TANF) cash assistance, Supplemental Security Income (SSI), or state-funded General Assistance are categorically eligible for SNAP. The state option of broad-based categorical eligibility also allows for the modification of some SNAP eligibility rules and has resulted in the vast majority of states not utilizing an asset test. **Data:** In FY2011, SNAP had an average monthly participation of approximately 44.7 million individuals in 21.1 million households. In FY2010, average monthly participation was 40.3 million individuals in 18.6 million households. Although this information is not yet available for FY2011, for FY2010, nearly half (47%) of participants were under age 18, another 8% were age 60 or older.	$78,300, not including $1,856 for Puerto Rico, Indian reservations, American Samoa, and the Northern Marianas, and not including TEFAP commodities.

Table 1. (Continued)

Authorizing Legislation / Federal Administrative Entity	Program Information	FY2012 Funding (in millions)[a]
The Emergency Food Assistance Program (TEFAP)		
The Food and Nutrition Act, Section 27 and The Emergency Food Assistance Act, Section 204(a) (7 U.S.C. 2036 & 7508(a)) / Administered by USDA-FNS	**Description:** Provides food commodities (and cash support for distribution costs) through states to local emergency feeding organizations (e.g., food banks/pantries, soup kitchens) serving the low-income population. **Eligibility:** States designate local emergency feeding organization recipients and establish income standards for individual eligibility. **Data:** Information on the number of recipients or the average value of benefits under TEFAP is not available.	$308
Community Food Projects Food and Nutrition Act, Section 25 (7 U.S.C. 2034) / Administered by USDA National Institute of Food and Agriculture	Competitive grants to nonprofit organizations for programs that improve access to locally produced food for low-income households. Eligibility for grants will vary according to request for applications.	$5
Commodity Supplemental Food Program (CSFP)		
Agriculture and Consumer Protection Act of 1973, Section 4(a) (7 U.S.C. 612c note) / Administered by USDA-FNS	**Description:** Provides supplemental monthly food packages (valued at approximately $25 a month) to lowincome elderly persons in projects located in 39 states, the District of Columbia, and several Indian reservations. **Eligibility:** Elderly persons (age 60+) who have access to a local CSFP project and household income below 130% of the federal poverty guidelines as well as women, infants, and children with income below 185% of the federal poverty guidelines. (States are prohibited from allowing dual participation in both WIC and CSFP.) **Data**: In FY2011, average monthly CSFP participation was 588,000 individuals. Approximately 569,000, or 97%, of the participants were over the age of 60.	$177
Fresh Fruit and Vegetable Program (FFVP)		

Authorizing Legislation / Federal Administrative Entity	Program Information	FY2012 Funding (in millions)[a]
Russell National School Lunch Act, Section 19 (42 U.S.C. 1769a) (expanded in Section 4304 of the Food, Conservation, and Energy Act of 2008 (P.L. 110-246) / Administered by USDA-FNS	**Description:** Provides grants to schools to purchase fresh fruit and vegetable snacks to be provided during the school day. **Eligibility:** Program is nationwide in select schools. States are required to select elementary schools in which 50% or more of the students are eligible for free or reduced price meals. Priority is placed on schools where the highest proportion of children are eligible for free and reduced-price meals. **Data**: Information on the number of FFVP recipients is not available.	$137[b]
Senior Farmers' Market Nutrition Program		
Food, Conservation, and Energy Act of 2008 (P.L. 110-246), Sec. 4231 (7 U.S.C. 3007) / Administered by USDA-FNS	**Description:** Provides grants to participating states to offer vouchers/coupons to low-income seniors that may be used in farmers' markets, roadside stands, and other approved venues to purchase fresh produce. **Eligibility:** Income eligibility criteria are established by states. **Data:** In FY2010, approximately 845,000 individuals in 42 states, the District of Columbia, Puerto Rico, and seven Indian Tribal Organizations received annual SFMNP vouchers/coupons worth an average of $33.	$21

Source: Prepared by CRS using USDA and P.L. 112-55 appropriations data.

a. For more information regarding FY2012 appropriations, including FY2012 funding as compared to FY2011, please see CRS Report R41964, *Agriculture and Related Agencies: FY2012 Appropriations*, coordinated by Jim Monke.

b. This is an approximation of FY2012, since the available amount is based in part on April 30, 2012, Consumer Price Index information. Also, general provisions in appropriations laws, P.L. 112-10 and P.L. 112-55, altered the amount of available FFVP funding.

Table 2. Overview of WIC and Child Nutrition Programs

Authorizing Legislation / Federal Administrative Entity	Program Information	FY2012 Fundinga (in millions)
Special Supplemental Nutrition Program for Women, Infants, and Children (WIC)		
Child Nutrition Act, Section 17 (42 U.S.C. 1786) / Administered by USDA-FNS	**Description:** Provides supplemental, nutrient-rich foods; nutrition education and counseling; and breastfeeding promotion and support to low-income women, infants, and children. WIC benefits are redeemable for a list of nutrient-rich foods specific to the participant's eligibility category and medical needs (for example, foods specifically recommended for an anemic pregnant woman). These foods are specified in USDA-FNS regulations, although state agencies may further specify. **Eligibility:** Pregnant, postpartum and breastfeeding women, infants, and children up to age five with household income at or below 185% of the federal poverty guidelines may be WIC eligible. Applicants must be individually determined to be at "nutritional risk" by a health professional and must meet state residency requirements. Applicants may also be categorically eligible based on receipt of TANF cash assistance, SNAP, or Medicaid. (States are prohibited from allowing dual participation in both WIC and CSFP.) **Data:** In FY2010, an average monthly total of approximately 9.2 million individuals participated in WIC— 4.9 million (53%) were children, 2.2 million (24%) were infants, and 2.1 million (23%) were women.	$6,620
WIC Farmers Market Nutrition Program		
Child Nutrition Act, Section 17(m) (42 U.S.C. 1786(m)) / Administered by USDA-FNS	**Description:** Provides grants to participating states to offer vouchers/coupons/EBT to WIC participants that may be used in farmers' markets, roadside stands, and other approved venues to purchase fresh produce. **Eligibility:** Women, infants over four months old, and children who are certified to receive WIC Program benefits or who are on a waiting list for WIC certification are eligible to participate in the FMNP.	$17

Authorizing Legislation / Federal Administrative Entity	Program Information	FY2012 Fundinga (in millions)
	Data: In FY2010, approximately 2.15 million WIC participants in 45 states and several Indian Tribal Organizations received annual FMNP benefits worth an average of $21 per year.	
School Breakfast Program (SBP)		
Child Nutrition Act, Section 4 (42 U.S.C. 1773) / Administered by USDA-FNS	**Description:** Provides federal cash assistance for elementary and secondary schools that provide breakfast to school children. Federal subsidies currently range from about 25 cents to $1.80 per meal (depending on the type of meal/snack and the income of the recipient, with subsidies higher in Alaska and Hawaii). Total amount of assistance is based on the number of free, reduced-price, and paid lunches served. **Eligibility:** Household income must be at or below 130% of the federal poverty guidelines for children to receive a free meal, above 130% and below 185% of the federal poverty guidelines for children to receive a reduced price meal. Direct certification allows household eligibility based on participation in SNAP, TANF, or FDPIR (Food Distribution Program on Indian Reservations). **Data:** In FY2010, an average of 11.7 million students participated each school day; 8.7 million received a free breakfast, 1.0 million received a breakfast at reduced price, and 1.9 million received a paid meal.	$3,320b
National School Lunch Program (NSLP)		
Russell National School Lunch Act (42 U.S.C. 1751 et seq.) / Administered by USDA-FNS	**Description:** Provides federal assistance, in the form of cash and commodities, to elementary and secondary schools that provide lunch to school children. Federal subsidies currently range from about 25 cents to $2.80 per meal (depending on the type of meal/snack and the income of the recipient, with subsidies higher in Alaska and Hawaii). Total amount of assistance is based on the number of free, reduced-price, and paid lunches served.	$10,200b

Table 2. (Continued)

Authorizing Legislation / Federal Administrative Entity	Program Information	FY2012 Funding[a] (in millions)
	Eligibility: Household income must be at or below 130% of the federal poverty guidelines for children to receive a free meal, and above 130% and below 185% of the federal poverty guidelines for children to receive a reduced price meal. Direct certification allows household eligibility based on participation in SNAP, TANF, or FDPIR. **Data:** In FY2010, an average of 31.7 million students participated each school day, 17.6 million received a free lunch, 3.0 million received a lunch at reduced price, and 11.1 million received a paid lunch.	
Summer Food Service Program (SFSP)		
Russell National School Lunch Act, Section 13 (42 U.S.C. 1761) / Administered by USDA-FNS	**Description:** Provides federal cash assistance and some commodity foods to local public and private nonprofit "service institutions" running summer youth programs, camps, or other recreation sites that serve low-income children during their summer break or during lengthy school-year breaks. Sites may be schools, camps, community centers, and other organizations. Sponsors receive per-meal/snack subsidies as well as assistance with operating costs. **Eligibility**: At a participating site, free meals/snacks are served to all children under age 18. **Data:** In FY2010, summer meals were served at over 38,000 sites to approximately 2.3 million children and youth.	$402[b]
Special Milk Program		
Child Nutrition Act, Section 3 (42 U.S.C. 1772) / Administered by the USDA-FNS	**Description:** Provides public or nonprofit schools or child care institutions that do not participate in other federal meal programs with a per-half pint reimbursement for part of the cost of milk served to children/students.	$13[b]

Authorizing Legislation / Federal Administrative Entity	Program Information	FY2012 Fundinga (in millions)
	Eligibility: Any child at a participating school or half-day pre-kindergarten program can receive milk through the Special Milk Program. Children may either buy milk or receive it free, depending on the school's choice of program options. **Data:** In FY2010, approximately 6.2 million half-pints of milk were subsidized through the Special Milk Program.	
Child and Adult Care Food Program (CACFP)		
Richard B. Russell National School Lunch Act, Sec. 17(o) (42 U.S.C. 1766(o)) / Administered by the USDA-FNS	**Description:** Provides cash subsidies to participating child care centers, family day care homes, afterschool programs, and non-residential adult-care centers for the meals and snacks they serve to children, the elderly, and chronically disabled persons. In child care centers and non-residential adult-care settings, per-meal/snack subsidy payments are the same as those for school meals and child care centers. Family day care homes are reimbursed according to a tiered system. Federal subsidies currently range from about 25 cents to $2.80 (depending on the type of meal/snack and the income of the recipient, with higher subsidies in Alaska and Hawaii). **Eligibility:** *(Adult services)* Elderly (age 60+) or chronically disabled persons attending participating nonresidential adult-care centers. Both for-profit and nonprofit centers are eligible to participate. Adults are eligible for free or reduced meals based on income guidelines that are the same as in school meals programs. *(Child care centers)* Children's eligibility for free and reduced-price meals and snacks is the same as for school meals programs. *(Day care homes)* There is no requirement that meals and snacks be served free or at reduced price. Instead, the homes receive a subsidy for every meal served; the size of the subsidy is based on whether the home is a Tier I or Tier II home. Tiering is based on the lowincome status of the child care provider or the community in which the provider is located.	$2,830b

Table 2. (Continued)

Authorizing Legislation / Federal Administrative Entity	Program Information	FY2012 Funding[a] (in millions)
	Data: In FY2010, the average daily participation of children and adults was approximately 3.4 million. Of the 3.2 million children served, approximately 2.4 million were in child care centers and 850,000 were in family day care homes.	

Source: Prepared by CRS using USDA data and P.L. 112-55 appropriations data.

a. For more information regarding FY2012 appropriations, including FY2012 funding as compared to FY2011, please see CRS Report R41964, *Agriculture and Related Agencies: FY2012 Appropriations*, coordinated by Jim Monke, pp. 61-71.

b. Approximately $1.2 billion in FY2011 funding is for commodity procurement ($900 million), administrative costs, studies, and evaluations across multiple child nutrition programs (school meals, summer food service, CACFP, special milk). This funding is not reflected in the per-program totals on this table.

Table 3. Overview of Older Americans Act (OAA) Nutrition Programs

Authorizing Legislation / Federal Administrative Entity	Program Information	FY2012 Funding (in millions)
Congregate Nutrition Program		
Older Americans Act, Title III, Part C, Subpart 1 (42 U.S.C. 3030e) / HHS-AOA	**Description:** Provides meals to seniors in settings such as senior centers, schools, and adult day care centers. Offers social services such as nutrition education and screening, nutrition assessment, and counseling at meals sites. Provides seniors with opportunities for social engagement and volunteerism. **Eligibility:** The following groups are eligible: (1) persons age 60 or older and their spouses of any age; (2) persons under age 60 with disabilities who reside in housing occupied by seniors where meals are served; (3) persons with disabilities who reside at home with, and accompany, seniors to meals; and (4) volunteers. **Data:** In FY2009, 92.5 million congregate meals were served to just under 1.7 million participants.	$440

Authorizing Legislation / Federal Administrative Entity	Program Information	FY2012 Funding (in millions)
Home Delivered Nutrition Program		
Older Americans Act, Title III, Part C, Subpart 2 (42 U.S.C. 3030f) / HHS-AOA	**Description:** Provides meals to seniors who are homebound. Offers services such as nutrition screening and education, nutrition assessment, and counseling. **Eligibility:** Persons age 60 or older and homebound and their spouses of any age. May be available to individuals who are under age 60 with disabilities if they reside at home with the homebound senior. **Data:** In FY2009, 149.2 million home-delivered meals were served to about 880,000 participants.	$217
Grants to Native Americans: Supportive and Nutrition Services		
Older Americans Act, Title VI, (42 U.S.C. 3057c) / HHS-AOA	**Description**: Provides for the delivery of supportive and nutrition services comparable to services provided under Title III (i.e., congregate and home-delivered meals) to older Native Americans. **Eligibility**: Older individuals who are Indians, Alaskan Natives, and Native Hawaiians. **Data:** In FY2009, 2.1 million congregate meals were served to 46,000 participants and 2.5 million homedelivered meals were served to 21,000 participants.	$28
Nutrition Service Incentive Program (NSIP)		
Older Americans Act, Title III, Part A, Sec. 311 (42 U.S.C. 3030a) / HHS-AOA	**Description:** Provides funds to states, territories, and Indian Tribal Organizations to purchase food or to cover the costs of food commodities provided by USDA for the congregate and home-delivered nutrition programs. Funds are allotted to states and other entities based on each state's share of total meals served during the prior year. Most states choose to receive their share of funds in cash, rather than commodities.[a]	$161

Notes: The FY2012 Consolidated Appropriations Act (P.L. 112-74, Division F, Section 527) applies a 0.189% across-the-board rescission on most Labor-HHS-Education items, including OAA and AOA items. The FY2012 funding figures do not reflect this rescission. For more information on programs and funding under the OAA, see CRS Report RL33880, *Funding for the Older Americans Act and Other Administration on Aging Programs,* by Angela Napili and Kirsten J. Colello; for more information on OAA nutrition programs, see CRS Report RS21202, *Older Americans Act: Title III Nutrition Services Program,* by Kirsten J. Colello.

a. In FY2010 (the year for which the most recent data are available), nine states chose to receive a portion of their share of the nutrition services incentive funds in commodities: Connecticut, Delaware, Idaho, Iowa, Kansas, Massachusetts, Montana, Nevada, and Oklahoma. The FY2010 value for these commodities was $3.4 million, see http://www.obpa.usda.gov/30fns2012notes.pdf, pp. 30g-70.

Source: Prepared by CRS based on appropriations legislation and committee reports; program data from the Administration on Aging, AGing Integrated Database (AGID) at http://www.agidnet.org/.

HHS-AOA PROGRAMS

The Department of Health and Human Service (HHS), Administration on Aging (AOA) administers domestic food assistance programs authorized under the Older Americans Act (OAA). These programs provide formula grants to states, U.S. territories, and Indian tribal organizations to support congregate and home-delivered meals to older Americans.[17] AOA also administers the Nutrition Services Incentive Program (NSIP), which provides funds to the same entities to purchase food for these programs. While OAA's nutrition programs provide food assistance in the form of a prepared meal to older individuals living in the community, the stated purpose of the program is not only to reduce hunger and food insecurity, but also to promote socialization, as well as the health and well-being of older individuals.[18] **Table 3** provides details on the HHS-AOA programs, including eligibility, services provided, and funding.

Older individuals who meet certain income and other requirements may also be eligible for other domestic food assistance programs administered by USDA, such as SNAP, the Senior Farmers' Market Nutrition Program, and the Commodity Supplemental Food Program (CSFP). While the senior nutrition programs are administered by AOA, there continues to be program coordination between AOA and USDA. At the federal level, states and other entities may choose to receive all or part of their NSIP allotments in the form of USDA commodities.[19] Obligations for NSIP commodity procurement are funded under an agreement between AOA and USDA.[20] At the state level, states and tribal organizations may collaborate with USDA programs such as CSFP, and can administer the adult component of the Child and Adult Care Food Program (CACFP), which provides meals in adult day care settings.[21] Moreover, other services funded under OAA may provide outreach and education to older individuals about available benefits and programs, such as SNAP and CSFP.

Congress has reauthorized and amended the OAA numerous times since it was first enacted in 1965. The last OAA reauthorization occurred in 2006, when Congress enacted the Older Americans Act Amendments of 2006 (P.L. 109-365), which extended the act's authorization of appropriations through FY2011. Thus, the authorization of appropriations for most OAA programs, including the senior nutrition programs, expired in FY2011. However, Congress has continued to appropriate funding for FY2012 activities. The 112th Congress may consider reauthorization of the OAA. In doing so, the committees of jurisdiction are the Senate Health, Education, Labor, and

Pensions (HELP) Committee and the House Education and the Workforce Committee.

End Notes

[1] There are additional federal programs that may provide food or meal assistance but these programs fall outside of what is typically considered to be the domestic food assistance programs. For example, while the early childhood education program, Head Start, may provide funds that go, in part, to providing meals, Head Start is not considered a food assistance program and is not included here. Similarly, emergency disaster relief programs administered by the Department of Homeland Security may in part provide sustenance as part of disaster recovery, but those programs are also not included in this overview.

[2] National Research Council, *Food Insecurity and Hunger in the United States: An Assessment of the Measure*, Washington, DC, 2006, pp. 23-51, http://www.nap.edu/catalog.php?record_id=11578. As a result of these findings, USDA now measures "low food security" and "very low food security," not hunger.

[3] Alisa Coleman-Jensen, Mark Nord, and Margaret Andrews et al., *Household Food Security in the United States in 2010*, U.S. Department of Agriculture, Economic Research Service, ERR-125, September 2011, http://www.ers.usda.gov/Publications/ERR125/.

[4] USDA-ERS website, "Food Security in the United States: Measuring Food Insecurity," http://www.ers.usda.gov/ Briefing/FoodSecurity/measurement.htm.

[5] Alisa Coleman-Jensen, Mark Nord, and Margaret Andrews, et al., *Household Food Security in the United States in 2010*, U.S. Department of Agriculture, Economic Research Service, ERR-125, September 2011, http://www.ers.usda.gov/Publications/ERR125/.

[6] U.S. Government Accountability Office, *Domestic Food Assistance: Complex System Benefits Millions, but Additional Efforts Could Address Potential Inefficiency and Overlap among Smaller Programs*, GAO-10-346, April 2010, pp. 51-53.

[7] The Community Food Projects are administered by the National Institute of Food and Agriculture (NIFA).

[8] See also USDA-FNS website, "USDA Food and Nutrition Service Regional Offices," http://www.fns.usda.gov/cga/ contacts/regioncontacts.htm.

[9] USDA-FNS SNAP Program Development Division, *Supplemental Nutrition Assistance Program: State Options Report*, Ninth Edition, November 2010, http://www.fns.usda.gov/snap/rules/Memo/Support/State_Options/9- State_Options.pdf.

[10] "Commodity" or "commodities" in the context of food assistance is broader and distinct from the term used to describe corn, wheat, soybeans, etc. in the context of commodity support programs such as described in CRS Report RL34594, *Farm Commodity Programs in the 2008 Farm Bill*, by Jim Monke.

[11] For more on the procurement of USDA foods, see CRS Report RL34081, *Farm and Food Support Under USDA's Section 32 Program*. For more information on FNS's distribution of commodities, please see USDA-FNS website, Food Distribution Programs and Services, http://www.fns.usda.gov/fdd/programs/default.htm.

[12] USDA-FNS website, "A Short History of SNAP," http://www.fns.usda.gov/snap/rules/Legislation/about.htm.

[13] Gordon W. Gunderson, USDA-FNS Website, "The National School Lunch Program: Background and Development," http://www.fns.usda.gov/cnd/lunch/AboutLunch/ProgramHistory_4.htm.

[14] USDA-FNS's Farm-to-School Initiative is described on the agency website: http://www.fns.usda.gov/cnd/f2s/. Further discussion of related policies can be found in CRS Report R42155, *The Role of Local Food Systems in U.S. Farm Policy*, by Renée Johnson, Tadlock Cowan, and Randy Alison Aussenberg.

[15] For more information on the Omnibus Farm Bill, please consult CRS Report RS22131, *What Is the "Farm Bill"?*, by Renée Johnson and Jim Monke.

[16] The Fresh Fruit and Vegetable Program, described in the table, was passed and financed by the 2008 farm bill program. It amended the Russell National School Lunch Act—a statute typically reauthorized elsewhere and in the jurisdiction of the House Education and the Workforce committee.

[17] The Older Americans Act (OAA) statute defines "older individual" as an individual aged 60 and older. For more information on programs and funding under the OAA, see CRS Report RL33880, *Funding for the Older Americans Act and Other Administration on Aging Programs*, by Angela Napili and Kirsten J. Colello. For more information on OAA nutrition programs, see CRS Report RS21202, *Older Americans Act: Title III Nutrition Services Program*, by Kirsten J. Colello.

[18] 42 U.S.C. 3030e.

[19] The Nutrition Services Incentive Program (NSIP) was originally established by the OAA in 1974 as the Nutrition Program for the Elderly and administered by USDA. Congress transferred the administration of NSIP from USDA to AOA in 2003. In 2006, pursuant to P.L. 109-365, Congress rescinded states' option to receive commodities. However, in 2007, this option was reinstated through P.L. 110-19 (effective April 23, 2007), which authorized the transfer of NSIP funds from HHS to USDA for the purchase of commodities and related expenses.

[20] Most entities choose to receive their share of funds in cash, rather than commodities. In FY2010, nine states chose to receive a portion of their share of the nutrition services incentive funds in commodities: Connecticut, Delaware, Idaho, Iowa, Kansas, Massachusetts, Montana, Nevada, and Oklahoma. The FY2010 value for these commodities was $3.4 million, see http://www.obpa.usda.gov/30fns2012notes.pdf, pp. 30g-70.

[21] U.S. Congress, Senate Special Committee on Aging, *Seniors Going Hungry in America: A Call to Action and Warning for the Future*, 110th Cong., 2nd sess., March 5, 2008, S.Hrg. 110–597 (Washington: GPO, 2008), p. 8.

INDEX

#

A

B

C

G

H

I

J

K

L

M

S

T

U

V

W